The Door of Last Resort

Critical Issues in Health and Medicine

Edited by Rima D. Apple, University of Wisconsin–Madison, and Janet Golden, Rutgers University, Camden

Growing criticism of the U.S. health care system is coming from consumers, politicians, the media, activists, and healthcare professionals. Critical Issues in Health and Medicine is a collection of books that explores these contemporary dilemmas from a variety of perspectives, among them political, legal, historical, sociological, and comparative, and with attention to crucial dimensions such as race, gender, ethnicity, sexuality, and culture.

For a list of titles in the series, see the last page of the book.

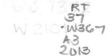

The Door of Last Resort

Memoirs of a Nurse Practitioner

Frances Ward

Rutgers University Press

New Brunswick, New Jersey, and London

Library of Congress Cataloging-in-Publication Data

Ward, Frances, 1950–

The door of last resort : memoirs of a nurse practitioner / Frances Ward.

p. ; cm. — (Critical issues in health and medicine)

Includes bibliographical references and index.

ISBN 978–0–8135–6053–3 (hardcover : alk. paper) — ISBN 978–0–8135–6054–0 (e-book)

I. Title. II. Series: Critical issues in health and medicine.

[DNLM: 1. Ward, Frances, 1950– 2. Nurse Practitioners—United States—Autobiography. WZ 100]

610.73'72069092—dc23

[B]

2012023498

A British Cataloging-in-Publication record for this book is available from the British Library.

Visit our website: http://rutgerspress.rutgers.edu

Manufactured in the United States of America

For Norbert

Contents

Preface

I was born a first-generation American to immigrant Scottish parents who settled in Kearny, New Jersey. From a diachronic perspective, my life as nurse and nurse practitioner was grounded in my early growth in this town. Maturing in a loving home shaped by the values of hard-working immigrant British parents, I enjoyed the luxuries of American higher education. As a student, I was a sponge. With education and experience, I immersed myself over time in unique events in distinct contexts, with dreams of an equitable health care system. Synchronically, certain tropes emerged in time, evidenced in behavioral outcomes; patterns of power relationships—equality, dualisms, reasoning, and valuing—evolved, invariably influencing what I live for. Perhaps more a blurred genre than either memoir or autobiography, my narrative recounts a life as a first-generation participant in the dismantling of medical autocracy in the United States—and the establishment of an alternative: the care of patients on their terms, in their context.

Over Time

The location of two Scottish manufacturers in Kearny—the Clark Thread Company and the Nairn Linoleum Company—cloaked the town in British values of hardiness, work productivity, and frugality. No one believed in the American dream more than my father. A highly skilled ship's carpenter in Scotland, in his early years in the United States he was termed a "Mick," mistaken as just another Irish immigrant looking for work. Once a member of the carpenters union, however, he had regular employment and benefits. Born in Dumbarton, Scotland, he was one of twelve children, completing the fifth grade in school. He married my mother, Frances, also from Dumbarton; but, as he wryly said, *she was from the other side of the tracks.* Also one of twelve, her family was engaged in the whiskey and liqueur trade; she completed high school and became a beautician. A British loyalist, she joined the Royal Army in World War II, becoming a front-line jeep driver. When the war ended, they came to the United States and married, eager for a new life.

My sister, Maureen, was born in 1948 and I was born in 1950. Living in Kearny with Scottish values, we were a close foursome. Schoolwork came first; phones were for business, not idle chatter; no television on weeknights; dinner at 4:30 P.M. after my father came home from a construction site; and play was outside, with pinky balls, jump ropes, and adventures in the Meadowlands. I'd walk into Newark to my favorite bookstore, where I bought Russian novels with saved bus fare money. We spent summers on the beach in Ocean Grove, beginning the day after school closed until Labor Day; my father worked in Kearny during the week and joined us on weekends. Time for work, time for play—and the ethic creed: If something is worth doing, it is worth doing well. I watched my mother roll saved pennies once her change jar was full. While summers in Ocean Grove depleted their savings for a home, they wanted my sister and me to enjoy summers away from the city. Only in retirement did my parents purchase their small dream home in Florida. At the end, they had plants, a lemon tree, jalousie windows, and air conditioning. New Port Richey was their home until my father, James Francis Ward, died five years after their move.

Rutgers—Into Newark

After my Catholic grammar and high school education, my life seemed to take on limitless potential in 1968 when I entered Rutgers University College of Nursing in Newark. From a sheltered Scottish environment to the swirling chaos of Newark, one year after the race riots—amid activist efforts of Students for a Democratic Society, the National Organization of Women, civil rights, Black Power, and the anti-Vietnam War movement—I achieved a stellar academic record, all the while stringing love beads, painting peace symbols, and sympathizing with all efforts at equality on any front. My father, a quiet man with pro-freedom fighter, anti-Crown inclinations, had shaped my thinking. I watched and listened to all events on the Newark campus between 1968 and 1972, the year I graduated with my Bachelor of Science degree. At Rutgers I felt the value of America's Declaration of Independence. Freedom of speech. Equality for all, including women and minorities. And health? Do not all Americans warrant quality health care?

Equally influenced by my stoic army mother, I obtained my first nursing position after graduation at the East Orange Veterans Administration Hospital (VAH) in East Orange, New Jersey. The reverence for veterans was paramount at the VAH; under the military ethos there, I was known as Nurse Ward. When I asked ambulatory patients on my oncology unit to help other less mobile patients with daily activities, I consistently heard a "Yes, Ma'am!" Embedded in an institution with a clear mission and exceptionally detailed scopes of practice for all employees, I learned how to care for patients as well as manage large, forty-bed units with minimal staff. Policies and procedures, numbered and unnumbered memoranda from Central Office in Washington were part of my day. My structured British background enabled me to fit into this system. Career advancement in nursing was available at the VAH; nursing positions were regularly published, each with educational and other requirements clearly outlined. In my early career, I enjoyed advancement from registered nurse in oncology, then on to intensive care; subsequently, I clicked into new roles as Clinical Nurse Specialist, and then, as Patient Education Coordinator. All actions at the VAH seemed to focus on one entity—duty to the veteran.

At the VAH I learned my drive to compete. Within six months at the VAH, I realized that to compete for advanced titles in the system, I needed more education. I looked to New York. Columbia University? No, too stodgy, too steeped in its own history. New York University? I was sold in one visit. Even the buildings exuded energy, color, vibrancy. I envisioned reading a book at the historic Washington Square Park, drinking my hot chocolate from the neighborhood Gristede's grocery. At Rutgers, I was a very good student; at NYU, I learned to think. I became confident at NYU. There was no thought you couldn't think; you simply crafted rationale to defend it. Faculty walked into classrooms and conversed with graduate students, who ardently absorbed the flavor and content of the discussions. Taking the PATH train from Harrison to New York City, I traveled from 1973 to 1981 earning a master's and then enrolling in doctoral courses at NYU on a part-time basis and working full-time, first at the VAH and then at Seton Hall University College of Nursing in South Orange, New Jersey.

I was thrilled to be a faculty member at Seton Hall. It was within walking distance from my home in the same town. Situated on a beautiful campus, with the Carolyn D. Swartz College of Nursing building constructed in 1973, Seton Hall nestled into its host community as a major face for South Orange, the Pirates commanding loyalty from local residents. It was a comfortable environment, but I was not matched well for it. As I increasingly questioned my world, fueled by my mentors at NYU, I became uncomfortable with the expected compliance demanded at this private, religious institution. It was a constraining environment, dogmatic in tone. When I left Seton Hall for a position at Rutgers University College of Nursing in Newark, I learned the culture of a public, research university.

In my five years at Rutgers University, I advanced from instructor to assistant professor, with an appointment to the Graduate School in Newark. My experiences at NYU deeply influenced my teaching at Rutgers: more constructs, less content; more inquiry, less dogma. A university for those who sought to excel, Rutgers was a road as diverged as any I had imagined. I learned the essence of the academy at Rutgers: the high stakes of tenure, the value of research and publications in the tenure process. As a young assistant professor, I taught students nursing care at Saint Michael's Medical Center, just a few blocks from the university. Always passionate about clinical care, and very proud of my expertise in acute care, I worked part-time at the medical center to assure my continued competency. Weekends at Saint Michael's, weekdays at Rutgers, evenings at NYU. It was a full life, with husband and children. I was awarded my PhD in nursing in 1982 while still an eager young assistant professor at Rutgers University. I was too busy for any ceremony of robes. During an evaluation session, my chairperson noted that I shouldn't waste my time with students in the clinical courses. Couldn't I find someone else to do my clinical coursework? I recall being angry. Nursing is a clinical discipline, and I was (and am) an expert clinician. I wanted to mentor my students at Saint Michael's; I thought of this as the most important aspect of my work. A tenure-track faculty appointment—with its ultimate promise of the award of tenure—seemed contrary to the essence of my discipline. It was an uncomfortable reality, even as I was on my way to successfully achieving the coveted goal.

I resigned from Rutgers after five years to return to the VAH for a short period. Rutgers had been a home with clear goals and missions, but I had grown inquisitive in the past years and now was restless, even in an institution I greatly admired. After a while, a colleague at the VAH encouraged me to respond to an advertisement for the position of chairperson for the department of nursing at the School of Health Related Professions at the University of Medicine and Dentistry of New Jersey (UMDNJ) in Newark. Curious for years as to why UMDNJ did not have a nursing school as one of its units, given its status as the state's only Academic Health Science University, I responded without hesitation. I was their only respondent—itself, a curious fact, but one that did not deter me from interviewing for the position. The president's goal: to have all health-related professions as part of the university community. When he had become the university's leader in 1970, he closed the hospital's diploma school, founded in the mid-1880s. Since that time, he wanted to establish academic nursing programs, undergraduate, graduate, or both. It seemed a simple matter. He was correct. It was a simple matter, given his enthusiasm, the resources he committed, and the wide base of support he offered. Never imagining I would be writing about all this ages later, I took that road.

A Room of One's Own

It was at UMDNJ that my Scottish work ethic singularly assured outcomes. While I gained confidence at NYU, I found my voice at UMDNJ. As a clinician in a health sciences university, I learned nursing's contribution to health care delivery, primarily by comparison and contrast to the disciplines of medicine, dentistry, and the various allied health professions. My niche was clear; my profession had a necessary place in care delivery. I also learned about courage as I moved forward professionally. After establishing the University's School of Nursing in 1992 and becoming its first dean, I matriculated in our nurse practitioner program and became an adult primary care nurse practitioner in 1998, working part-time in the University Hospital's emergency department in addition to my administrative role. As a political as well as an academic institution, UMDNJ flourished through legislative efforts. As the nation's shortage of primary care providers became pronounced in the late twentieth century, I became involved in legislation to name nurse practitioners as primary care providers. Through my relationship with New Jersey State Senator Wynona Lipman, I crafted language for her bill seeking prescriptive authority for nurse practitioners. My policy and administrative background informed my historical research into nursing's history in New Jersey, an effort that informed my appreciation for the influence of power, politics, and legislation in nursing practice.

My twenty-three years at UMDNJ passed in a seeming blink of an eye. Once I had returned to the classroom from administration in 2002, I became restless again. While I found engagement with students rewarding, I also found myself dulled by the constancy and repetitiveness of teaching, even online teaching. And, although I have a robust research agenda that involved the establishment of reliable and valid instruments to measure learned helplessness and community living skills, I missed administration. When approached by Temple University College of Health Professions to serve in its David R. Devereaux endowed chair of nursing, I took a pied-à-terre in Philadelphia and moved into a new, old role.

Temple, a large comprehensive public research university, is located in North Philadelphia, surrounded by a host community marked by poverty and poor health indices. All over again, here was déjà vu. My experiences at establishing a school of nursing in New Jersey would be very valuable at Temple; at least, so I thought. Temple's nursing program had its roots in a diploma program begun in 1893, the year of the Chicago World's Fair, an exciting time of change and educational advancement. That was also the year when the American Society of Superintendents of Training Schools of Nursing, the predecessor to the current National League for Nursing, was organized. Once it was transitioned to a Bachelor of Science in Nursing degree program in 1967, however, nursing simply became one of several health profession programs constituted as departments in a newly established College of Health Professions. After an enthusiastic faculty agreed with me to implement a new shared faculty governance model, they subsequently revised curricula to stay ahead of the health reform curve, virtually transforming programs from a hospitalist orientation to a primary health care model.

I elected to retire from Temple in 2012. Telling all this with a sigh, I will now watch change there from a distance.

Tropes over Time

In fall 2011, my elderly father-in-law was hospitalized in Louisiana with a severe infection and renal failure after having had bilateral knee replacement surgery a few months earlier. His surgeon, a regionally acclaimed expert in orthopedics, left surgical rounds of his hospitalized patients to his nurse practitioner, Darlene. My husband and I were instructed to talk with her in the hospital when we wanted updates on my father-in-law's status. My husband spoke with the charge nurse: Can you please page my father's nurse practitioner for us? A quizzical look, a raised eyebrow. Her answer was delayed, as if by the strangeness of the request. We don't page nurse practitioners. In fact, we don't even know their names.

Louisiana, New Jersey, Pennsylvania. Irrespective of state, nurse practitioners have remained relatively invisible as primary care providers in the delivery system. Despite the widespread acclaim that nurse practitioners represent a critical solution to the inadequate number of primary care providers across the United States, not a great deal is known about their scope of practice, their education, and their philosophical orientation to primary care. As a branch of the profession of nursing, the largest single health care discipline in the country, nurse practitioners—advanced practice nurses—are recognized by health insurers as primary care providers. Significantly, indices of current popular books exploring problems of the U.S. health care system do not reference nurse practitioners. Equally significant, books written for popular audiences by nurse practitioners about nurse practitioner practice—advanced practice nursing—are rare. Two such books come to mind. Laurel Thatcher Ulrich, a Pulitzer Prize–winning early American historian, provided readers with an accounting of a midwife's work and life in her 1990 study *The Life of Martha Ballard, Based on Her Diary, 1785–1812*. Julie Fairman, a nurse historian, provided a historical analysis of the nurse practitioner movement in *Making Room in the Clinic: Nurse Practitioners and the Evolution of Modern Health Care* (2008). One is a late-eighteenth-century documentary study, the other an early-twenty-first-century historical analysis. This is all we have. Nurse practitioners' silence about themselves and their practice is patently obvious. It is a silence cloaked in nursing's historical models and value dualisms.

How do nurse practitioners think? How do they describe primary care? Do their answers to these two questions differ significantly from those of other providers? Jerome Groopman explored *How Doctors Think* in his popular 2007 book. Groopman explained physicians' cognitive shortcuts—or heuristics—as the core of flesh-and-blood decision making. Physicians' thoughts-in-action, their clinical reasoning patterns that determine diagnoses and treatment plans, are deemed by Groopman as evidence-based techniques that are the foundation for medical thinking. Medical education provides the patterns for recognition of diagnoses, if not the actual heuristics. Education is the foundation; time at task provides heuristics. As Michael Crichton noted about Groopman's book in his article "Where Does It Hurt?" (*New York Times,* April 1, 2007), Groopman recognizes the value of patients' stories and their involvement in care, yet "medical education has regarded communication skills with an indifference that approaches contempt. It's unscientific."

While a book with the title *How Nurse Practitioners Think* has yet to be published, nursing's early roots in monasticism have cultivated a sentimental societal image of a nurse as the vehicle for nurturing activities attendant to the alleviation of suffering as mediated by the physician. With its embedded requirements of absolute obedience, constrained voice, and limited expertise, monasticism shrouded the discipline of nursing in invisibility. Over time, *nurse* has become synonymous with hospital, given that nurses are the workforce needed to provide care and assure hospital cost recovery. As noted by Charles Rosenberg in *The Rise of America's Hospital System* (1995), nurses settled on a public image of devotion and sensitivity rather than discipline-specific cognitive skills in order to acquire public acceptance in the late nineteenth century. Such settling has resulted in a systemic failure so deep that even the classification in the Integrated Postsecondary Education Data System for my specialization—adult nurse practitioner—is misleading. The inclusion of adult nurse practitioner as an illustrative example under the title Adult Health Nurse/Nursing, rather than as a separate entity itself, creates noise in the signal.

Signs signify what resides in cultures. A sign links to that which it signifies. I posit that neither the word "nurse" nor the phrase "nurse practitioner" have signifiers that uniquely convey shared understanding among Americans. Without clearly unique scopes of practice appropriate to the level of education among those holding the registered nurse (RN) license, the sign "RN" defaulted to a cultural image of a caring, gentle female emulating mothering, nurturing behaviors. Bernice Buresh and Suzanne Gordon in their 2006 book, *From Silence to Voice: What Nurses Know and Must Communicate to the Public*, have described the image of nursing and how that image would be redefined, if nurses want to take an active role—and responsibility—in changing this image. Since nurse practitioners must be, first and foremost, nurses, the cultural ethos surrounding nurse practitioners—their roles and their cognition—are grounded broadly in our culture's view of nursing. The earliest nursing model—that of virtue—signified "nurse" as a composite of values emanating from this paradigm that was firmly established in the late nineteenth century. The virtue model continues into the twenty-first century; however, its impact is diminishing, gradually having been replaced in the later twentieth century by transitional gumbo—virtue blended with discipline-specific functions consistent with our country's focus on science, technology, engineering, and mathematics. Post-*Sputnik*, post–Admiral Rickover. Virtue was still necessary, but not sufficient.

How nurse practitioners think, their cognitive patterns involving their practice, is deeply influenced by their education as nurses. Undergraduate nursing curricula address the nursing care needs of societies as encompassing health needs, both physical and psychiatric, enmeshed, among other factors, in a rich interaction of cultural and spiritual beliefs, housing and other environmental factors, socioeconomic status, educational achievement, family support, and community resources. Undergraduate students are encouraged to assess patients' needs, their resources, their desire for healthier lifestyles, and their capacity to achieve such improvements. Patients are at the center of nursing care, making decisions based on information given to them from providers, including nurses and nurse practitioners. Diagnoses belong to patients; once informed, their wishes for care are to be honored. Thus, the nurse practitioner's heuristics, if they were explored under the title *How Nurse Practitioners Think*, emanate from graduate education providing foundations of clinical reasoning alongside courses in epidemiology, anthropology, perception, culture, and other disciplines that explore humans in the context of their environment. Conversations about patient-centered health homes versus physician-centered medical homes highlight the differences between nurse practitioner and physician thinking.

These differences shift power relationships. In nurse practitioner cognition, the patient has power. In physician cognition, the physician has control and power. Should a patient not conform to a physician's plan of care, she may be viewed as noncompliant. Should a patient be unable to conform to a plan of care mutually agreed upon earlier by the patient and nurse practitioner, the plan is changed; the patient is not blamed for failure. In hospitals, nurses conform to rules generated by physicians and hospital administrators; there, nurses care for physicians by complying with medical orders. In primary care, nurse practitioners construct management plans consistent with patients' needs, resources, capacity for adherence, and overall goals. All courses in a nurse practitioner's broad undergraduate nursing education, as well as in graduate courses, are prerequisite for safe primary care delivery.

In the early twenty-first century, nurse practitioners blend virtue and something else in a transitional state. Currently, some nurse practitioners aim to practice as replacements for physicians; they emulate medicine's model. Accepting and embracing the complexity of patients' contexts, others practice differently. Acceptance of context is a line in the sand, a trope of an evolving nurse practitioner model. Context is an essential externality embedded in the practice of nurse practitioners. Patient-centeredness mandates the embrace of context. The simple recognition of a patient's economic status influences a nurse practitioner's prescribing practices. Prescriptions for generic medications, along with instructions to purchase medications at local pharmacies with low-rate monthly charges, are part of a practice cognizant of context. Discussions emerge on the value of continuing education in order to improve confidence, meet goals, improve self-worth, and alleviate depression. Ignoring context may create burdensome costs in care delivery, in that negative externalities—such as poverty, lack of knowledge, poor housing conditions, ignored addictions, and others—may delay positive health outcomes and impact quality of life. My patient with hypertension, anemia, and bipolar disease is reminded that she has a voice—and the privilege to use it.

As nurse practitioners move from the virtue model through the transitional model to a new heuristic of practice based on context, other tropes are noted. Shifting control to patients in a patient-centered, context-driven model is an act of disruption in a postmodern, global era. The modern-era medical practice—complete with centralized authority and illness orientation—may continue indefinitely until other tropes of a new heuristic are more universally endorsed. One such trope is self-efficacy. Albert Bandura, a prominent psychologist known for the development of social cognitive theory, defines self-efficacy as the belief that one has the capability to perform in a way that positively affects one's life. As nurse practitioners embrace the new heuristic of practice based on context, the uniqueness of their primary care behaviors will become increasingly self-evident. No longer skirting a hazy, hybrid practice existing in the borderlands between medicine and nursing, their confidence is enhanced. Gloria Anzaldúa, a prominent scholar of Chicano cultural theory, described a borderland as an unusual place demanding hybridity—a conscious flexibility allowing invisible survival without legitimate power.

Abandoning the cloak of virtue in exchange for self-efficacy also involves abandoning the secondary gains attendant to either the virtue or transitional model. Hybridity can generate complacency, a conscious choice to have peaceful days without power, but great predictability. Walking away consciously from hybridity is a disruptive act. To be disruptive is to be accountable. Disruptive acts interfere with obligation dualism, the dualism that traps nurses in both the virtue and the transitional models to coexist within competing tensions of obligation to self (individualism) versus obligation to society (collectivism). Such competing tensions conspire to trap nurse practitioners in an oppressed, but comfortable, performance ethic of low risk. Nancy J. Hirschmann, a political scientist, suggested in her 1992 book, *Rethinking Obligation: A Feminist Method for Political Theory*, that postmodern duality structures a world of paired opposites that provide individuals with identities not of their own construction that are highly oppressive. Reflection on such value dualisms reveals the importance of a heuristic model of nurse practitioner practice based on context. In place of contemporary health care, a new scope of practice deeply embedded in patient-centeredness brings into play another trope: accountable self-regulation. As virtue and hybridity are replaced with the new heuristic, the hazy fog surrounding nurse practitioner practice lifts. A scope of practice is established framed in nursing, not borrowed from other fields. Self-efficacy and self-regulation are welcomed as the risks associated with visible practice in the delivery system are no longer threatening.

My experiences as a nurse practitioner versed in policy, history, practice, and education allow me to describe in this book the possibility of a heuristic model of practice based on context. We are moving toward this model, but we are not there yet. Once it is embraced by a majority of nurse practitioners, our patients will profit—as will the delivery system itself.

The Door of Last Resort

Chapter 1

Bread Is Not Sugar

Uninsured and underinsured urban residents receive primary care in starkly contrasting health facilities—from expensive, state-of-the-art hospital emergency departments staffed by hospitalists to neighborhood health centers staffed by nurses. In the latter, nurse practitioners use basic diagnostic tools to offer primary care services. The focus is on patient context. Here, I take my stand. Through narratives of my experiences as an adult nurse practitioner in both an urban emergency department and in rudimentary nurse-managed urban health centers, I give voice to the scope of practice of a nurse practitioner. Such stories reveal how nurse practitioners think. Beyond cognition, the stories help me describe the intricate network of relationships that exist among providers in various community-based organizations. This web of relationships sustains the financially fragile yet critically needed safety net that binds us together in the service of a common humanity. The stories offered in chapter 1 establish questions that will be explored further in other chapters: Who owns the language of health care? Is health care patient centered or provider centered? And, with their focus on the patient's context, just how disruptive are nurse practitioners in a health care system that reimburses for the singular cost of illness?

*

I arrived early at the health center. The large plastic clock with the drug name Protonix written in yellow and blue across its face reported the time as 7:30 A.M.

While patients did not typically arrive earlier than 9 A.M., today was different. Darlene, my petite thirty-five-year-old African American patient with
hypertension and Type 2 diabetes mellitus, left a message the day before that
she wanted to see me today. Her phone message was tremulous, halting, and
almost fearful in tone. She would come over to see me in the morning right
after her shift at work. Sorting bed linens and preparing laundry carts for use
on patient units in a nursing home during the day, Darlene was a night shift
worker. She also helped with other tasks, calling herself a go-fer. She would
be off work at 7 A.M. and see me around 8 A.M. Invisible, she was one of those,
as David K. Shipler reminds us in *The Working Poor* (2004), who did not have
the luxury of rage.

Camden Was Context

A lifelong resident of Camden, New Jersey, Darlene lived with her father and
four siblings in public housing. I first met her about a year earlier, when she
stopped at the health center to have her blood pressure checked. She had dis-
covered the center through a flyer left on a pew in her church. Her pressure
was high—Stage 2 hypertension based on criteria published in 2003 by the
Joint National Committee on the Prevention, Detection, Evaluation, and Treatment of High Blood Pressure, an arm of the National Heart, Lung, and Blood
Institute. She complained of headaches and feeling very tired. Exhaustion was
a luxury. Her physical examination was unremarkable, except for her blood
pressure. Her history revealed a different story. "Pressure," as she called hypertension, had gone badly for all of her siblings. Two had asthma. Her mother
had died from sugar, with her father currently on the kidney machine for pressure and sugar. One brother had suffered a stroke about one year earlier, and
it was now hard for Darlene to take care of her father at home. A spot check
of her urine revealed a dark green color indicating approximately 500 mg urinary glucose excretion—an abnormally high amount. I became concerned that
Darlene had diabetes.

Darlene was the family's matriarch, dealing with health, legal, and other
issues swirling around in her always tense home. A high school dropout and
unemployed all of her adult life until recently, Darlene was not on public welfare and did not have Medicaid health benefits. She said she lived with her
family, a statement that implied a tangled web of codependencies for income,
housing, food, and anything left over constituting daily existence. In exchange
for her maintenance, Darlene took care of the family's needs, from caring for her
severely disabled brother to running errands. During her initial visit, I treated
Darlene for Stage 2 hypertension, giving her a thirty-day supply of a thiazide

diuretic that I had available through pharmaceutical samples. I also give her a prescription for blood work to determine if she had diabetes. Following my instructions, Darlene had her blood work taken at a local medical center's outpatient department. The results, confirming my suspicion that she had diabetes, were sent to me at the health center.

The bill was sent to her.

I added an oral antidiabetic medication to her regimen. Since her blood pressure was not adequately controlled with a diuretic, I added a second antihypertensive drug to her regimen, giving her one I had available through pharmaceutical samples.

Management of her hypertension and diabetes was trivial compared to management of her hospital laboratory bill. Although Darlene would cut a deal with the hospital finance office to start monthly payments of ten dollars to eradicate her debt, she quickly fell into arrears, her failure to meet a commitment devastating her pride. Against her family's wishes, she had taken her present job at the nursing home, which included health benefits. *I am the only one in my family that has ever had a job, that I can remember*, she told me. *The nursing home staff really depends on me*, she proudly stated. With a photocopy of her plastic benefits card on file, I was then able to prescribe the diagnostic work-up that I knew was appropriate, including evaluation of her cholesterol, renal function, electrocardiograph, and more. With data and evidence-based guidelines in hand, Darlene and I managed her chronic health problems together, bringing both her diabetes and hypertension under control.

Now, a year later, Darlene's phone message worried me. I reviewed her chart and prepared my single examination room for the day. She was unusual. Employed full-time with health benefits, Darlene could receive the full scope of management accorded others with health insurance. Mostly everyone else who would walk through the door that day was either employed but uninsured—our working poor—or unemployed and without welfare and Medicaid benefits. Others were illegal workers, fearful of deportation; they came to the center for help with acute problems. A few with health insurance routinely came to the center as a step on their way to (*What should I say again?*) or from (*What did he mean?*) their doctor. I rephrased and decoded. Darlene had named my collaborating physician as her primary care provider, and since I had a collaborative agreement with him—such an agreement is a requirement for nurse practitioners to practice in New Jersey—I routinely managed her at the center. Ideal, I believed, given that I had established the Camden center several years earlier to extend primary care delivery in the city. Darlene provided evidence that this system was working.

My emergency room background from years spent in Newark had trained me to make three-second assessments. When she walked in, it was clear that Darlene was very tired. Dark circles under her eyes, her shoulders drooping, she sank into the little dark blue plastic chair—my Tupperware chair as I termed it—beside the exam table, too tired to speak. Perhaps I could grant her the luxury of exhaustion.

Her family obligations plus her job were so very, very tiring, she said. *I go to work tired, and I get home even tireder.* Her family wanted her to quit her job; they needed her more at home. More. She was torn, afraid to go home, fearful that they would not let her rest. More. She needed to talk, to validate that what she was doing was not selfish. I assured her that working and caring for her health was not only unselfish, but also responsible behavior. We reviewed her diabetic diet and medications. Darlene smiled broadly as she told me that she had paid off her hospital laboratory bill. She left to go home to sleep. More exhaustion.

Darlene's grip on the priority of health was tenuous, easily challenged by the more pressing priorities in her life—family responsibilities, family pressures—to serve others rather than to care for herself, an ever selfish act. I was the single, fragile link encouraging her to continue her defiant behavior of survival.

As Darlene left, two other people were waiting outside my office to be seen. My two-room center—an office and one exam room—were located at the end of the first-floor corridor in an old two-story building owned by the Camden County Council on Economic Opportunity. Originally a county library, the gray stone building was worn and dilapidated with age, in need of much repair. Serving as a central home for the administration of social and welfare programs offered by the council, many employees hustled daily through the building, coordinating services for their poor clients—one step ahead of the swirling themselves. Employees had a choice—either opt for health benefits, with the mandatory copay, or receive more money in their paychecks. Most opted for the larger salary.

Gloria was one such employee. Like Darlene, she had hypertension. Unlike Darlene, Gloria was obese. Every Wednesday—the center was open only on Wednesdays—Gloria would get weighed and have her blood pressure checked. When she first started coming to me for care, Gloria weighed 275 pounds. Given her 5 foot, 4 inch height, Gloria had a Body Mass Index (BMI) of 47.2, Class III obesity—40.0+ BMI extreme obesity—according to the National Heart, Lung, and Blood Institute's Obesity Education Initiative, a major effort launched in 1991 to reduce the national prevalence of overweight. Gloria was quite leery of drugs, given her past long history of intravenous drug use. Now, as Gloria wryly said, *I am only addicted to food.* Knowing that obesity was associated with diabetes and high blood pressure, Gloria sometimes wondered out loud if her health was better served when she was addicted to cocaine. Today we negotiated weight management and hypertension drugs. We would go slow and paced with dietary changes—beginning today with a diet diary—and drug management. Gloria agreed to take a thiazide diuretic for her blood pressure, believing that she could use the water loss, since her ankles seemed swollen to her lately. She was very afraid to begin any changes in her lifestyle, fearing that she might return to cocaine if she had to decrease her food intake in addition to taking medications.

We talked about how food is metabolized, with excess calories converted to fat and stored. Carbohydrates in bread, I noted, are broken down in the body, causing an increase of sugar. I was kind, Gloria concluded, but not especially bright. *Miss Fran*, she told me in a voice filled with gentle reservation, *bread is not sugar.*

Our conversation continued, and Gloria and I agreed on a singular action regarding weight: she would keep a diet diary for one week. The diary was to be reviewed the following week, with changes in her daily eating habits that she could regard as reasonable. Admitting that a loaf of bread a day might be a lot of bread, she thought that she might even start by taking one less slice of bread per day. While Gloria needed a cardiovascular and diabetes evaluation, what she needed more was management by a registered dietician. I was pleased that Gloria was willing to try a diuretic and to chart her daily intake—both for only a week. Ultimately, however, she did not have faith in the health care system—*Aren't most of us in Camden fat with high pressure and sugar diabetes?*—but she did have faith in those who worked in the Camden County Council on Economic Opportunity gray stone building, formerly the library.

As mentioned earlier, our center was open every Wednesday. I had established the center in 1999, when I was the founding dean of the University of Medicine and Dentistry of New Jersey School of Nursing. At first it was open every day and managed by a registered nurse who provided basic primary health care, including primary promotion and education activities. Eventually, nurse practitioner faculty from the school rotated at the center, expanding services to include primary care management. With family practice physicians from the School of Osteopathic Medicine serving as collaborative practice partners, the health center became a site for both care delivery and student clinical experiences. As state budgets for higher education became tighter, the staff diminished at the center; by 2004, only one nurse practitioner faculty provided services one day a week. My service at the center was computed as part of my faculty workload, rather than being an income generating practice that would bring money back to the School of Nursing. Here was sophisticated volunteerism, social service rendered in capitalistic terms.

I had toyed with the idea of closing the center. It was impossible for me to do that, however. As the founding dean who had returned to the faculty role in 2002 before social good and capitalistic pursuits collided in the pages of the *Newark Star-Ledger* in 2005, I felt stubbornly responsible to make the role of nurse practitioner work at the center. Closing it was certainly an option, perhaps the most realistic, practical option from a financial perspective. I held tenaciously to demonstrating the value of nurse practitioner practice in underserved areas serving residents with poor health indices. So I stayed, as much an act of defiance as an act of commitment.

The defiance mandated committed partnerships. Fortunately, the director of the council continued to view the center as a needed health service, complementing the social and welfare programs offered by his employees. He did not charge us rent or overhead costs. The few supplies we routinely ordered—recurring clinical supplies, glucose and cholesterol monitoring devices, scales, tuberculosis skin-testing materials, and the like—were obtained from an interest account of an endowment obtained from a large philanthropic organization. In Camden, health care was delivered a step ahead of the swirl, rendered with sample pharmaceutical supplies, referral phone calls to community partners, and Wal-Mart discount prices on generic drugs—four dollars for a thirty-day supply of a generic medication. Here was health care mediated by patients' chief complaints as understood within the context of family histories and lifestyle choices. Formalism was a luxury; Camden was context.

Since most of the council's programs were grant funded, including management of Camden County's Head Start Programs, I conducted free annual physical examinations mandated for continued employment. One of the components of the annual examination was tuberculosis (Tb) skin testing. Through our endowment interest account, I ordered purified protein derivative (PPD) skin tests from a local vendor—who developed a strong relationship with the center, personally delivering supplies in his car rather than having them potentially lost—and began providing this test to comply with requirements for annual Tb screens.

The PPD Tb skin testing quickly proved to be problematic. Once the test is administered, the site of administration must be read forty-eight hours later to determine if the patient has a positive or negative reaction. Since the center was only open all day on Wednesdays and Saturday mornings from 9 A.M. to noon, skin tests could not be read forty-eight hours later at the center. To offer Tb skin tests, a partner was needed. The council, in addition to managing Head Start Programs, also ran the Urban Women's Center, offering apartments and training to women in need. This site, located only three blocks from the health center, employed a professional staff willing to be trained in reading Tb skin test results. After extensive training in tuberculosis, skin testing, and evaluation of test results, PPD tests could be offered both on Wednesdays and Saturdays at the health center. Patients could have their test results read by trained staff at the Urban Women's Center, with results forwarded to me—at no cost—for follow-up. In turn, a relationship with the city's department of health was developed; thus, I sent any patients with positive results there for further evaluation and management. Slowly, a loosely constructed network of partners was developed with whom, and through whom, I could extend services.

As Gloria returned to her office, affirmed in her belief that I was kind but dull, I ushered the second waiting patient into the exam room. She was new to me, and very intriguing. Florence, a middle-aged African American female, with a brilliant smile, bizarre, colorful clothing, and excessive makeup, told me in a firm, vibrant voice that she was glad to see that I was finally open for business. She had undergone cardiac surgery a few weeks earlier and, upon discharge, was told to follow up at Camden County Council's health center on Broadway, with me, on Wednesdays. Florence was fifty-two years old, receiving income, under the table, from caring for children in her home. Hypertensive, with coronary artery disease and several weeks postcardiac revascularization surgery, Florence still had angina (though much less than before) and new complaints of leg pain when she walked more than a block or two. I was stunned that Florence was sitting in my Tupperware chair seeking follow-up care. She had no health insurance and no appreciable income. She had never received public welfare, surviving on part-time jobs and on health care delivered in emergency rooms when her home remedies no longer helped her. Whether experiencing dental pain or chest pain, Florence either walked into her local hospital's emergency department or called for the city's ambulance to take her there. Given that her local hospital was one of the state's regional trauma centers associated with a medical school, Florence received state-of-the-art acute care services, paid for by New Jersey's program of charity care, legislated by Public Law 1997, Chapter 263. Upon discharge, she typically relied on her family's medical practices—herbs, candles, and rest—and her faith in God to help her convalesce and return to health. In the phrase Mary Abrams used to describe health beliefs in the journal *Social Science and Medicine,* after a while Jesus would fix it.

Florence had now run out of her chest pain medicine (nitroglycerine) and her legs were bothering her, so she came to me that day for a prescription and some advice. *Here's what I need,* Florence said, *nitro and make my legs better.* Firm, confident, businesslike. Florence represented something new to me—an uninsured patient with multiple, complex problems, discharged from an academic health sciences center for continuing management at a local, neighborhood, one-day-a-week center.

More committed partners were needed.

I cultivated CAMcare, a federally qualified health center (FQHC) offering services in southern New Jersey at seven locations that provided primary care to insured and uninsured patients. One CAMcare location, on Federal Street, is within blocks of the health center. As an FQHC, CAMcare provides health services to persons of all ages, regardless of their health insurance status or ability to pay. It provides a health care safety net program under the U.S. Department of Health and Human Services. After completing a complete history and physical examination on Florence, I called CAMcare, seeking an appointment for cardiology and vascular evaluation and management. One triage nurse—Steve—became my link to CAMcare. A full-time registered nurse at CAMcare, Steve accepted my FAXed documentation and provided Florence with a date for the evaluation she needed. In the meantime, I called the local Wal-Mart pharmacy to see if they had Isosorbide Mononitrate 60 mg extended release tablets available. The Wal-Mart four-dollars, thirty-day program is a valuable, critically needed option for all patients. Isosorbide Mononitrate is designed as a routine continuing drug to prevent angina attacks, not to alleviate acute chest pain. My local Wal-Mart pharmacy did have this medication in stock, and Florence left the center with a prescription to fill there, a referral for evaluation and management at CAMcare, and two drugs for management of her stage two hypertension. I gave her thirty-day supplies of amlodipine and hydrochlorothiazide from my stock supply of sample drugs obtained from two sources—drug company representatives and my colleagues' clinical offices at the School of Osteopathic Medicine. My collaborative physician's administrative coordinator, on a monthly or so basis, provided me with sample drugs to bring to the health center. Typically, I brought antihypertensives, antibiotics, antidiabetic, and heartburn medications, and asthma controller drugs back to the center. Since so few of my patients had prescription drug plans, pharmaceutical companies did not send representatives to the center; thus, my friendship with colleagues at the School of Osteopathic Medicine was quite important for my patients.

Florence clearly needed social services, particularly to help her enroll in public welfare and Medicaid. While the Camden County Council did provide social and assistance programs for the needy, no social workers were available to provide guidance. Eventually, I learned that the Camden County Board of Social Services, with headquarters on Market Street, again within walking distance of the health center, was a valuable partner. Florence was referred to the board for guidance, and soon did receive public assistance and Medicaid health insurance. In time, she and I negotiated with this system to help locate an additional source of financial support—the Supplemental Security Income, a federal income supplement program funded by general tax revenues designed to help disabled people with little or no income. Florence did receive supplemental income and a permanent pass for the city's buses. Florence's unstable cardiovascular status and her extremely poor vision, despite management both at the health center and CAMcare, entitled her to these resources. At first, Florence was reluctant to accept the supplemental income. She soon realized, however, that her new, expanded income—$800 more a month—provided her with enough money for rent, utilities, and food. She no longer needed to care for children in her home to survive.

Here's what I need: nitro and make my legs better.

Begun.

My last patient this same day was Netty, a seventy-two-year-old African American female who came to the center in the late afternoon in the company of her friend. Her friend was concerned. Netty didn't seem just right today. She was very tired, weak, and didn't seem to understand what was happening around her. When Netty was too weak to stand by herself, her friend brought her around the corner to the center. Was Netty going to be OK? Netty's blood pressure was 208/110; her friend confirmed that her pressure was usually high. Her neurological exam revealed right-sided weakness, inability to walk without assistance, facial droop, and slow, slurred speech. Netty did not have a history of stroke, only hypertension and arthritis. I phoned a new partner—the emergency department of the local academic health sciences medical center. I called for an ambulance and contacted the hospital, reporting that Netty would arrive with a presentation consistent with cerebrovascular accident—or stroke. The emergency room physician to whom I gave Netty's history was unimpressed. Are you sure it wasn't just a transient ischemic attack? Maybe I could give her some medication and attempt to bring the pressure under control in the center? I assured her that it was not safe for Netty to remain with me, and I ushered the ambulance away with Netty in it. Another lesson. When to, and not to, send a patient to the emergency department for evaluation and management. A prickly partner, but a partner nonetheless.

One day at the health center in Camden was more complex than my previous work as an adult nurse practitioner in a university hospital's fast-track emergency service. Interacting as a provider, a confidante, an advisor, and more, I found the work at the center exhilarating, and sometimes draining. The work demanded a willingness to view health as part of a broader system of interacting urban components—housing, transportation, and education. General welfare. Beyond hierarchy.

The Real ER

You've sewn before, haven't you?

That's what the emergency department physician said to me frantically as he turned his back on me, ready to bolt out of the little exam room in which a patient, writhing in pain and holding his torn right heel as it hung bloodily from his foot, desperately needed suturing. He had a gunshot victim on a gurney. As a nurse practitioner student I had sutured pig skin, cleanly, slowly, and in magnificent detail in a practice laboratory in the college. This was 8 P.M. on a Saturday night in University Hospital, Newark, New Jersey. My patient had been triaged to the fast-track service, a unit staffed by nurse practitioners established to manage the needs of less acute patients. Essentially, the fast-track service was the primary care provider for uninsured and underinsured residents in the local community—a large patient population. On a Saturday night, the very definition of primary care varied, given the nature of presenting complaints, number and types of trauma cases, and sheer volume of patients to be seen.

On another night, my patient might have been treated in one of the trauma sections of the emergency department—the big rooms, as we called them. Tonight was busy.

Despite the hour, the department was stunningly awake, with blinding lights, yelling staff, crying visitors, hallways and exam areas awash with sounds, odors, and debris strewn everywhere. To those at work, a controlled chaos; to others, a scene from a military battleground. *Turkeys, you've cooked turkeys, haven't you?* the attending physician asked me with a sense of stunning urgency. Yes, I had stuffed and cooked many a turkey in my life. Suddenly, I understood. If I enjoyed the privilege of working in this department, then I needed to participate fully, without hesitancy. *If you do the first stitch, then I'll do the rest*, I recall having said, even as I tugged the patient onto the stretcher and positioned the overhead light. See one, do one, teach one, an old motto alluded to in health professions education. Taking advice from Marta, a seasoned physician's assistant who also worked in the fast track, I gave the patient a local anesthetic and cleansed the wound—scrubbing with a Betadine surgical scrub brush until I was satisfied that the wound was clean. The patient, a young male unwilling to give details surrounding his trauma, was in his early thirties, with scars on his abdomen and evidence of old wounds on his legs. Encouraging me to take my time, *I'm in no hurry, and I'm safe here,* he closed his eyes and drifted to sleep as I sutured his heel. After receiving a tetanus toxoid booster injection—he couldn't recall when he had last received tetanus toxoid—and instructions on wound care and follow-up management in the medical clinic, he was discharged.

As my sutured patient was preparing to be discharged, the registered nurse asked if I had given him antibiotics, either sample medications or a prescription. It was an interesting question, revealing a common, and controversial, practice in wound care. Since he had no ostensible risk factors—he was not diabetic, was not HIV positive, was not immunocompromised—and the wound was exceptionally clean, I had not prescribed prophylactic antibiotics. The nurse was appalled, somewhat shaking my fragile confidence. Even as I relayed my rationale to her, I knew she was disturbed. Provider addiction to prescription antibiotics is astounding. As a novice practitioner expert only in the academics of primary care, I knew my decision was correct; however, the pressure from patients and providers alike to write prescriptions is burdensome. As a faculty person responsible for teaching nurse practitioner students about antibiotic management, I was wedded to the Centers for Disease Control's multiple twelve-step programs to encourage providers to give antimicrobials sparingly and only as warranted, all in an effort to halt antibiotic resistance. The pressure to prescribe antibiotics, however, is daunting, requiring a hardiness that grows only with time and confidence. Marta, my physician's assistant colleague, assured me that her scrub technique had never failed—as long as the patient didn't have risk factors, a good scrub and suture would suffice.

Guardedly confident, I approached my next patient, a young woman escorted by a cadre of staff and a police officer. Sobbing and disheveled, virtually held up by the police officer at her side, she blurted out *I've been raped!* My mind raced. Rape victims require specific examinations and collection of evidence, frequently used in court proceedings. In New Jersey, sexual assault forensic examinations are performed by licensed registered professional nurses trained to provide comprehensive care to sexual assault victims. Such a nurse, certified by the State Board of Nursing as a Forensic Nurse—Certified Sexual Assault (FN-CSA) after successfully passing both clinical and didactic examinations, is called upon to examine rape victims. Such a specialist had been notified by the triage nurse. My role was to obtain the patient's history of the present chief complaint and general medical history. Unable to find a quiet room conducive to interviewing, I placed the patient in a regular exam room in the fast-track area. Like all such exam rooms, by the end of a long Saturday it had the appearance of having been heavily used, with filled garbage cans and sharps containers, saline containers, intravenous fluids and angiocaths at the ready. Stark, metallic, and oddly austere in appearance. With my patient reclining on the exam table, still sobbing, and me in a chair at her side, I asked her to relay her story. As clinicians often begin when describing patients, I noted that she was alert and oriented times three; that is, oriented to time, place, and person. She described her attacker as a middle-aged white man who was really quiet. After at least several minutes during which she closed her eyes and rested, I mentally reviewed the next steps of her case, as in all such cases. It was critical that all evidence be collected properly in order to be considered admissible in court. I wrote my notes fastidiously, anticipating the arrival of the FN-CSA. As I was writing in the patient's record, she sat up and asked me if I knew how difficult it was to have sex with a dead person. As she continued describing her rape experience, I recalled advice that I had received during my initial education in nursing: *Do not confuse orientation status with contact with reality.* I switched referrals, seeking consult with the psychiatric crisis unit rather than initiating sexual assault protocols.

Still fairly new to the role of adult nurse practitioner, I wanted time to write my notes as I had painstakingly instructed students to do, and then to calmly usher in the next patient. But that is an unheard-of luxury in an urban emergency department, particularly on a weekend evening. A young male, escorted by two police officers, had been brought in from the local county jail for severe dental pain. He was febrile, tachycardic, and rocking back and forth in a chair, holding his left jaw with his hand. He had multiple dental caries, missing teeth, and widespread erythema and swelling in his lower left gum. One tooth, highly decayed, had fractured, and pus was oozing from the surrounding tissue. University Hospital is an academic health sciences center, with attending physicians and residents in oral-facial-maxillary surgery on call. Given that he had no allergies to medications, I asked the nurse to give him two injections: one Bicillin, an antibiotic, and the second, Toradol, a nonsteroidal anti-inflammatory drug commonly used for analgesia, anti-inflammation, and for pain relief. Surprisingly, the nurse refused, stating that I was also a nurse, she was busy, and I could give these medications myself. Marta and I exchanged glances. She and I had recently had a conversation about the relationships we had noted among some registered nurses and nurse practitioners. Some registered nurses refused to take orders from nurse practitioners or physician's assistants. Occasionally, tensions between registered nurses and those certified in New Jersey as advanced practice nurses—nurse practitioners, clinical nurse specialists, certified nurse midwives, and certified registered nurse anesthetists—bubble to the surface. In my case, I asked if she would give these medications so that I could call for the referrals to OMF, thus dividing our labor for efficiency. In practice, this tension is disarming, causing delays in care.

Nurses are sometimes described as a group who sometimes eat their young. Because they often oppress each other, they are easy prey.

On the other hand, the OMF group responded quickly to my referral. One of the many advantages of working in a fast-track service in an academic health sciences campus is the ready availability of professionals for referral and consultation. The patient was whisked away to a dental suite for evaluation and treatment, his chart moving with him. I found it oddly disconcerting that my dental colleagues, focusing on the patient, responded quickly and appropriately to my referral, whereas my nursing colleague had to be cajoled into working with me. Certainly in my past I had heard nurses sometimes speak negatively about nurse practitioners as mini-doctors, nurses who had abandoned their nursing roots and philosophy in exchange for a prescription pad.

My practice in the fast track heightened my awareness of the power of language and the perceived ownership of certain words: diagnosis, prescription, referral, consultation, even patient—words ostensibly owned by medicine and implying power and income. When used by nurse practitioners, some providers—nurses and physicians alike—assume a defensive position, guarding vigilantly their turf as defined by language, with all of its rich implications. This ownership of language effectively shifts the focus from the patient to the provider, reinforcing roles and power relationships. An exhausting reality. A hybrid role built on a registered nurse license and extending primary care delivery through advanced training in diagnosis and management, the nurse practitioner, I accepted sadly, must be emotionally strong to manage the complexities of the practice. Here were Gloria Anzaldúa's borderlands, described in *Borderlands: The New Mestiza/La Frontera* (1999). *La Frontera* requires the mestiza consciousness of flexibility and endurance, a hatred of hierarchy and a love of hybridity.

While professional relationships may at times be fragile, particularly intra-professional relationships, the work with patients in the fast track was thrilling. The last patient I treated after my dental patient was wheeled away was a young male who had sustained a rather deep laceration over his left eyebrow in a gang fight. He was sixteen—all energy, like a cat that had recently tangled with a blue jay and won, feathers still caught in his whiskers. He was pacing, talking rapidly about *getting the guy who did this to me!* Frequently, facial lacerations may be referred to plastic surgery, particularly with young patients. Such surgeons, however, were in the big room, engaged in caring for more extensive cases. I remember feeling calm; after all, just a few hours earlier, my heel trauma patient had been discharged without adverse effects. I conferred with my mentor, asking advice on the type of suture to use. Taking his advice, I sutured my young patient's laceration slowly, realizing that his facial appearance would be forever marred if he developed an extensive scar or infection. He was very cooperative, helping hold an overhead light in a certain position when I called upon his help. But he was too afraid of injections to accept the tetanus toxoid, so he was charted as refusing medical advice. Before he was discharged, we had time to talk. Had he completed high school, I asked? No, but he said he was good in math and some day, he did want to work with computers. We briefly spoke of community colleges, specifically Essex County College in Newark. Health, according to the World Health Organization, is not merely the absence of disease or infirmity, but rather a state of complete physical, mental, and social well-being. On a prescription, I wrote: *Go to Essex County College.*

Amazingly intermeshed with education, health is a complex construct. And, in urban neighborhoods, health may not be a priority, especially as poverty deepens. In a high-rise, low-income community adjacent to the hospital, the housing council had approved a one-room community health center run by the nursing faculty and students in the late 1990s. At first not deemed necessary—after all, wasn't the hospital right next door?—this health center became important to the residents of the community. Managing common acute and chronic health problems, this center enabled patients to go to the hospital only for emergency care. At the center, however, patients owned their health and negotiated with the nurse practitioners for the care they wanted and were willing to accept, such as one, but certainly not two, drugs for hypertension management. And, some therapeutic lifestyle changes—perhaps more exercise, dietary improvements, smoking cessation, or others—advocated by the National Heart, Lung, and Blood Institute and the American Heart Association—were accepted, while others were rejected. Perhaps they presented not the perfect picture of compliance, but patients agreed to well-negotiated regimens based on compromises to suit their preferences.

For years I worked in this environment as a full-time dean and part time as an adult nurse practitioner in the fast-track service of University Hospital. It was an exciting environment, a safe environment in which to learn primary care management. Always embedded in a team of providers, always able to turn right or left for guidance, the fast track provided a safe, diverse learning ground for understanding the common acute and chronic problems managed in urban settings. Each day I appreciated the resources available for medical, surgical, and trauma problems, the sheer amount of supplies expended daily in emergency departments. I frequently instructed patients to seek help at the intake area for applications to charity care, a state program to provide acute care to indigent, uninsured patients. I also began to recognize the lack of sophisticated delivery services for dental and mental care—D & M—two areas of care delivery that are left unmanaged in our delivery system. They frequently coexist among myriad other more demanding medical diagnoses for which technologies and diagnostics are available. Over time, I also noted that health care is commonly equated with hospital care; that acute illness management is an adrenalin rush for providers, teasing their critical diagnostic reasoning abilities; that lifestyle management is the harder regimen to engage in—it is easier for a provider to treat the complications of diabetes mellitus (hyperglycemia, coronary artery disease) than to change the lifestyles associated with poor outcomes (cessation of smoking, exercise, diet management).

After two years as a student in the fast-track service and four years as a part-time provider in it, I moved into community primary care in Camden. It was a sharp contrast to University Hospital in Newark; the two-room center was quiet, dull in appearance, poor in resources, but incredibly valuable in the neighborhood it served. Shifting from the hyper-vigilance associated with state-of-the-art diagnostics and interventions, the focus turned to patients—their complaints, negotiations on management regimens, and practical therapeutic lifestyle changes intended to inch slowly toward improved health indices.

I could never return to the emergency room, the hospital, and all they entailed. Beyond hierarchy, I took up residence in the interstices.

A Community of Broken Windows

In March 2004, I received a call from the director of the women's program at the Hispanic Family Center of Southern New Jersey, located in Camden. Did I want to offer a health fair at the Hispanic Center in March in honor of Women's History Month?

The call from Altie, the director, could not have come at a better time. The health center, previously staffed by UMDNJ's School of Nursing with a registered nurse and nurse practitioner faculty, now offered health services only one day a week, by me. Years earlier, an internal medicine colleague of mine in Newark said, in an aghast, exasperated voice, *You simply cannot do primary care in a one-room health center!* While I did not agree with him then, I now understood that what passes for primary care comes in a variety of sizes and shapes. In affluent communities, primary care is most frequently provided in large, ambulatory-practice locations with pastel interiors and soft music, a full array of on-site diagnostics, a small army of insurance billing agents and coders, and at least one appointment clerk. In urban centers with uninsured and underinsured residents, as well as illegal aliens, primary care is cobbled together through networks of care providers. Community-based organizations, committed to their local neighborhoods, string together services, generally through local, state, or federal funds and grants from philanthropic organizations. While primary care may not be delivered in a one-stop environment, it may be obtained through a series of steps taken in a community network.

As Altie and I explored how I might participate in her celebration of Women's History Month at the Hispanic Center, I began to feel my self-confidence return. Even as one person, it could still work. The health center would remain open. Conceptualizing the health center as central in a network of partnerships, I reoriented my view of my practice. Altie and I decided to offer a health fair at the Hispanic Center on March 9 to any clients receiving services that day.

How is a health fair evaluated? My past experiences with such events were mixed. On one hand, they were a terrible waste of time and supplies, with few people triaged appropriately for follow-up services. However, if organized with planned mechanisms for follow-up management, then such a fair might bring people into the system that might not otherwise seek care or be evaluated. Given that my funding was limited, I needed to target very specific services for the fair. First, what were the main health indices of the Hispanic population in Camden? A review of the New Jersey Department of Health data, in addition to findings included in the U.S. Department of Health and Human Services' *Healthy People 2010*, validated trends I was aware of from my own practice. Obesity, diabetes mellitus Type 2, metabolic syndrome, hypercholesterolemia, and hypertension. These were—and remain—the primary health problems faced by the community served by the Hispanic Center. These data guided my spending on supplies. Using the recommendations published by the United States Preventive Health Services Task Force, a professional group sponsored by the U.S. Agency for Healthcare Research and Quality, I zeroed in on screening for health problems that were most prevalent in the area. So I shopped, using my endowment interest account: blood pressure cuffs (adult and obese cuffs), a scale, tape measure (to measure abdominal girth and height), glucometer (to measure blood sugar), and cholesterol monitor. With these relatively inexpensive supplies, Altie and I managed forty-eight clients during my first day at the Hispanic Center. The majority of these clients were either overweight or obese, according to the published criteria on BMI, with many having a positive family history of diabetes. The majority also had enlarged abdominal girth, a factor considered relevant in the evolution of metabolic syndrome, a group of risk factors associated with coronary artery disease, stroke, peripheral vascular disease, and diabetes mellitus. And, while hypertension was not a major problem in this group, hypercholesterolemia was quite common. Additionally, many women complained of being frequently tired, with lethargy noted as a complaint among young adult females.

Our first health fair at the Hispanic Center resulted in one young female being sent to the local emergency room for severe hypotension with tachycardia and exhaustion, ten referred to their primary care providers for evaluation of their weight and cholesterol, and another ten given appointments with me for follow-up care at the health center. Of these ten, three were given prescriptions for one-month supplies of antihypertensive medications, the most prescribed drug being hydrochlorothiazide, a diuretic. One female was encouraged to see her primary care provider for evaluation for polycystic ovarian syndrome, given her physical signs and test results—overweight, acanthosis nigricans, and hypercholesterolemia. Additionally, in the context of high BMIs, the common complaint of tiredness intrigued me. With my remaining interest funds for that year, I purchased a HemoCue, an instrument to measure hemoglobin, a blood component that decreases with anemia.

This first health fair event with Altie, who marvelously orchestrated client flow and triage, providing a dedicated interpreter to help me, shifted my work at the health center. Altie and I decided to make the health fair a regular event at the Hispanic Center, with recruitment flyers and announcements circulated within the local community. Altie aligned staff members to perform specific functions during these events—one served as an interpreter, another managed data collection using a standardized patient form, a third determined patient flow and on-the-spot referrals—and successfully integrated this fair as a standard service. I provided her with reports from each health fair, including summary data of follow-up referrals, many of which were useful to her as she garnered grant support for her programs. At a subsequent event in 2004, forty-three clients were evaluated, the majority of whom were repeat clients from the first event. Obtaining regular data on blood pressure, cholesterol, glucose, weight, abdominal girth, and eventually, hemoglobin became an incentive for change in lifestyle. Of these forty-three clients, the overwhelming majority were obese with increased abdominal girth, and 23 percent had three major risk factors of metabolic syndrome, the precursor to diabetes mellitus, coronary artery disease, and peripheral vascular disease. And, my hunch proved correct.

Twenty-eight percent of these clients had low hemoglobin—that is, below a value of 12, indicating anemia—and another 28 percent had borderline values between 12 and 13, revealing risk for anemia. Many of the anemic patients were also obese. These data begged for therapeutic lifestyle interventions.

Where does a single provider begin in a culture marked by obesity, poor health indices, and low income? The issues were simply too big to consider as a single phenomenon. I needed to break the phenomenon down to a series of single variables, factors I could manage, outcomes I could evaluate simply and successfully. Low hemoglobin and *tiredness.* Low-hanging fruit? Clearly, improved diet is the most time-honored intervention for iron-deficiency anemia. Diets, however, are related to culture—and income. I therefore bypassed diet and visited Wal-Mart. Multivitamins with low-dose iron, such as the brand name Flintstones Complete, cost approximately six dollars for a sixty-day supply. Generic brands, from large warehouses such as Sam's Club, BJ's, and Costco, cost even less. I investigated low-cost foods high in iron—but low in cholesterol—and began an advocacy campaign for multivitamins with iron, lentils, peanuts, dried beans, raisins, chicken (baked, not fried), green leafy vegetables, and oatmeal. Given that tiredness was most pronounced among working mothers with small children, this program snowballed into family life, since female clients changed some aspects of their families' regular eating patterns as well. *What are these again? Raisins? Are they candy?* Raisins and fruit juice, rather than candy and soda, became my mantra. A visit to the Rutgers University Family and Community Health Sciences Cooperative Extension resulted in another partner—this program sent staff on site at specific locations to demonstrate cooking for healthy lifestyles. While certainly not unique, these efforts were significant, raising awareness of the relationship between how you feel and what you eat, while being cognizant of cultural preferences and income.

Over time, the health services at the Hispanic Center expanded to include tuberculosis testing, with training of the staff to read the skin tests and to forward results to me at the health center for follow-up if needed. The relationship established at CAMcare became quite significant for patients who required additional diagnostic evaluation, then returned to me for routine management at the health center. One client, Mercedes, a fifty-year-old female, was a recent immigrant to the United States, living with family in north Camden. Obese and diabetic, Mercedes was determined to get control of her health—and a job. Enrolled in the English as a Second Language class at the Hispanic Center, Mercedes began to learn English; she also took classes in basic computer skills. With the equipment available to me at the health center—my history-taking and physical examination skills, glucometer, cholesterol screening device, HemoCue, scale, and otoscope/ophthalmoscope—and my listening skills, Mercedes used her diet diary daily, evaluating her eating habits and weight loss weekly. She decided to visit me weekly, if only to validate her improvement and *to get*, as she said, *an A on my report card!* In one year, she had lost ten pounds, a tremendous improvement; while still in the BMI-territory of obesity, she had dropped from obese II to obese I category. Success. She purchased red nail polish for herself to celebrate her accomplishment.

Many of the clients serviced at the Hispanic Family Center had health insurance, either through Medicaid or their employer. What became apparent to me in time was a type of common substandard management of illnesses in this population. Frequently, I wrote referral notes to clients' primary care providers with suggestions for changes in their medical management. Perhaps a second drug to help lower the patient's Stage 2 hypertension, consistent with the Joint National Committee recommendations? Or, the introduction of an oral antihypercholesterolemia medication to control a client's total cholesterol, in addition to encouragement to *eat better.* Or, insulin for a diabetic patient who had been unsuccessfully managed with diet control and one oral antidiabetic medication? Complacency, an absolute acceptance of poor health indices in this population, and the endorsement of mediocre management for a rather silent, invisible population were the norm. For some clients managed by their primary care providers with substandard treatments, I encouraged a change of providers, often urging reassignment to providers in CAMcare, the federally qualified and federally funded health and migrant center in Camden. I encouraged the small number of clients with private health insurance to change their provider to my collaborating physician associated with the University of Medicine and Dentistry of New Jersey in Stratford, who had offices throughout South Jersey. In either case, the care would be improved, given the presence of teams, the visibility of patient outcomes, and the avoidance of overt greed. The idea of choice came as a surprise to many of these patients. One goal of the Hispanic Family Center, a comprehensive human services agency, is empowerment.

Empowerment is alarming to predators. Years earlier, when I was starting a small health service in a housing complex in Newark, a physician colleague said that he would gladly be my collaborating physician if I would give him half of all the money I made. There was no money to be made in an indigent population of uninsured residents; I didn't shake hands with him.

George L. Kelling and James Q. Wilson were correct in their 1982 theory: with broken windows creeps apathy and greed. Criminal invasion comes from many sources.

Within a year of starting to work alone at the health center in Camden, I was busy. The data were exciting; the results of effects from simple interventions were accumulating. Diet, simple exercises, changing providers, and routine visits for validation of success—all were means to an end in improving health indices. The School of Osteopathic Medicine decided to rotate student volunteers in family medicine to the health center on Saturdays to provide care to children. My colleagues also changed their curriculum to incorporate community health services as a rotation in the family medicine program.

The school of nursing began to value student experiences at the health center as well. My experiences with undergraduate nursing students at the center were not stellar, sad to reveal. Too many students were in a small space, left vaguely to my charge—irrespective of the patient services I was present to conduct. While I too preach see one, do one, teach one, it is impossible to do that with a fairly large group of students. The urban community, unlike the acute care hospital, is not as honored a location for attention to meticulous care, with students frequently opting out of real engagement. Like the community providers I had encountered in the neighborhoods of the Hispanic Family Center, students in community health rotations did not consistently demonstrate the commitment and passion required to positively impact residents' health status. Their love of hospitals and acute care continued to trump local neighborhood and community health services. The paradigm of health care delivery remains a modern-era phenomenon, with hospitals designated as the primary locus of care. Time at Camden was, perhaps, time not well spent, in students' minds.

Service in the Great Society

The letter from the Head Start director asked me to serve on the program's advisory council, a group providing guidance to the director on matters affecting the curriculum of the program, as well as the health and welfare of the children. In 2004, all of the twenty or so Head Start programs offered in Camden County were administered by the Camden County Council on Economic Opportunity (OEO), with its main office in the same building that housed the health center. The building was on the corner of Broadway and Royden Avenue, Camden. The executive director of OEO administered these programs, operating within federal guidelines for professional staff, curricula, and student requirements. OEO, established in 1965 as a private, nonprofit organization, had one goal: to use available resources to eliminate poverty as a destructive force in society— consistent with Lyndon B. Johnson's Great Society's dreams of imagined equality. Kidney machines, pressure, sugar, and the health of children were part of Camden's faltering health infrastructure.

Since one of my major contributions was to conduct the annual history and physical examinations, as well as tuberculosis testing, for Head Start employees, I had developed a relationship with the staff at the main Head Start office, located just three blocks from the health center. Many employees met their obligation to comply with the regulation for annual testing by scheduling physicals with me, irrespective of their health insurance status. I enjoyed doing these exams, which allowed me to understand the health concerns of the OEO community I served. Participating in the Head Start Program's advisory council was a natural commitment for me, one I thought reasonable.

I was stunned by the discussions held during my first advisory council meeting. To admit children to Head Start, documentation of compliance with health screening requirements needed to be met. Such screening included standardized assessment of speech, hearing, vision, physical examination for disability, and laboratory testing. Results of anemia and blood lead levels were required prior to including children in the program. Interestingly, these requirements were inconsistently met, even for children covered by health insurance. And, for parents of uninsured children, the health requirements posed a barrier—one that program staff often ignored, allowing needy children into the program without complete fulfillment of the requirements. Here was a no-win situation, circumscribing the powers of a rational mind, straight from Joseph Heller. However, the health center did have a HemoCue machine to measure hemoglobin, the particular lab value mandated to assess the presence of anemia in children. What I did not have was the ability to measure serum lead levels, but the New Jersey Department of Health and Senior Services did have a Lead Screening Program.

After a series of phone calls to various officials within the department, I eventually found a partner—the professional staff member who conducted the Lead Screening Program. If we collected the finger-stick blood samples from the children and express mailed them to him along with the appropriate paperwork, he would provide the lead evaluations. I placed my name on the paperwork as the responsible agent, representing the health center that collected the samples. The Head Start director supported the trainer program in which I instructed her staff collecting the finger sticks for lead testing. After a summer training program, we provided several all-day assessment programs in which staff collected lead finger sticks, in which I collected hemoglobin samples, and in which nursing students tested for tuberculosis by a skin test.

This partnership enabled the appropriate documentation of health assessment to be completed prior to the start of the program, thus ensuring compliance with regulations. The health manager at Head Start was the contact person who would initiate follow-up for any abnormal values returned from the state. The partnership with the Lead Screening Program was short lived, however, since my contact at the state level indicated that the processes were changed in his office, eliminating our arrangement. While free or reduced-cost lead screening continued to be available at other centers, the ease provided by the on-site program, conducted in the OEO building, increased compliance. In the complexities of life in the city, our program helped the very people targeted most by Head Start.

As the lead screening initiative, spurred on by my involvement on the advisory council, played out, the need for additional programming became evident. What are the signs that a child is anemic? What happens to the central nervous system when blood lead levels are elevated? What are normal versus abnormal behaviors in young children? What behaviors require referral or consultation with a health care provider? Such questions by members of the Head Start staff stimulated other instructional programming through the health center. Programs on the normal growth and development of preschool children, including normal behaviors, as well as programs illustrating the signs and symptoms of anemia and high lead levels were offered to staff. In a short period, my involvement in OEO's Head Start program had expanded from conducting employees' annual health assessments to instructional programs. Health required knowledge; knowledge was empowerment—a nascent goal of Johnson's original Great Society.

While working with Head Start staff was thrilling, my involvement came at a cost. My one-day-a-week participation in our school's health center had taken me away from my primary care specialization and led me more toward a global primary health care delivery orientation. Given my multiple partnerships— with Head Start, the Hispanic Family Center, and others—as well as my commitments to health education and care delivery, I now had less time to devote to seeing my patients. Nursing students' participation, although present, was minimal; and neither sustained nor of dependable quality.

I was compelled to recall that primary care is but one component of primary health care, which is a larger construct. In 1978, at the International Conference on Primary Care sponsored by the World Health Organization, the Declaration of Alma-Ata defined health—determined to be a state of physical, mental, and social well-being—to be a fundamental human right. The value-dualism between primary care practice and a more global orientation to primary health care had to be mediated within the framework of patient-centeredness.

If the integrated, complex system of primary health care coordinated through the school's health center was to continue, then others needed to become involved. I needed to determine my own priorities. Primary care or primary health care? To be certified as an adult nurse practitioner by the New Jersey State Board of Nursing was a career achievement, especially poignant given my past battles with medicine to obtain the privilege of diagnosing and treating patients. The battles were brutal, with language the key weapon. Who owned the patient? Who had the right to diagnose? After years of constant lobbying, nurses gained the right to engage in primary care through Chapter 377, *Laws of New Jersey*, 1991. One could never let one's guard down; sustained hypervigilance was required if nurse practitioners were to retain privileges won through legislation. Our academic graduate programs at the school prepared nurse practitioners to serve in various fields.

As I found myself, through necessity, moving toward delivery of primary health care in Camden, I realized that involvement of others within the school was needed. This involvement came through need, a common stimulus that drives change. As student enrollment in undergraduate programs increased, the need for more community health placements also increased. Undergraduate students in an accelerated baccalaureate program were assigned to the health center, under the supervision of a seasoned nursing faculty. These students participated in health fairs and screenings, as well as health education programs.

As students participated, I was able to provide more direct primary care, a role I now understand I coveted jealously. The network of partnerships in Camden—with community-based organizations, Head Start, OEO, CAMcare, and others—had grown to serve as a small safety net for some of Camden's residents. The rate-limiting factor to its growth and effectiveness was clearly the personnel dedicated to both primary health care and primary care. And given the likelihood that student involvement could not be considered predictable, the system of care that had evolved through partnerships might not be sustainable. Grants were certainly a possible way of offering services for a delimited time, similar to the sporadic involvement of students. But grants demanded assurance of sustainability—the very concept most likely to shift around unreliably in the delivery of health care to uninsured, underinsured, poor urban residents.

Meeting the demand for hypervigilance concerning physicians' moves to restrict nurse practitioner practice, compounded by worries over sustainable urban care to poor residents, takes energy. Movement between and among communities of health care providers—nurses, physicians, health centers—leads to hybridity, the uncertainty of a borderlands existence. It was a hard life to live alone.

For approximately two years, Darlene and I worked together to manage her health goals. Her hypertension and diabetes were now under control, with a medication and diet regimen that she accepted. She never was able to afford the luxury of rage. Eventually, I saw less of her. At first, I wasn't concerned. While her visits were less frequent, she did come in for evaluation prior to reissuing of prescriptions. But then her visits simply ceased. I asked another patient, her close neighbor, if Darlene was OK. The neighbor said Darlene was fired and had left Camden.

She wasn't sure where she had moved to, but she did say that Darlene left by herself, to start over.

Chapter 2

Health Care

Perspectives from the Street Level

At the Philadelphia's Mary Howard Health Center, my primary care practice deepened with immersion into the health care reimbursement system. Credentialed as a primary care provider by Keystone Mercy Health Plan and Health Partners, I became reimbursable. No longer a billable externality along with laundry management, my services to my Medicaid patients were reimbursed to the Public Health Management Corporation, the owner of a network of nurse-managed health centers in the city. With an administrative infrastructure emulating ambulatory physician practices embedded in manicured suburban landscapes, these federally qualified health centers are financially sustainable facilities. Caring for homeless patients at Mary Howard forced me to take a position on the value dualism deeply embedded in the U.S. delivery system: care of patients versus management of disease. Caring for patients from their standpoint, I intensified my definitions to include the possibility of negotiation and compromise at every turn. How risky to practice primary care with the patient at the wheel. How liberating to abandon disjuncture. Demands by insurance payers swirl at the boundaries of my practice. We are to focus solely on patients' chief complaints rather than their stated health needs. We are to follow the paramount mantra: No Margin, No Mission! Yet such demands themselves reveal the underutilization of registered nurses in the system, providers with a capaciousness of skill untapped in primary care delivery. Framed in the door of a nurse-managed health center is a physician, stating with exasperation that *you simply cannot do primary care in this place!* My experiences proved him

wrong, so very wrong. Balancing mission with margin, my work at Mary Howard helped me to understand nursing's unique contributions to primary care.

*

As I walked down South Broad Street in Philadelphia in August 2010, wide sidewalks steamy with heat, I felt light, sure, confident. I had an appointment with Tine Hansen-Turton, JD, chief executive officer of the National Nursing Centers Consortium (the Consortium for short), an organization of nurse-managed health centers serving vulnerable people across the country. The Consortium, headquartered in Philadelphia, is housed on the eighteenth floor of the Atlantic Building at 260 South Broad Street, just two blocks from City Hall. (A neighboring historic building—the Bellevue-Stratford, built in 1904—houses the Independence Foundation, a private, not-for-profit philanthropic organization also involved with nursing centers.) The Atlantic Building, located in the city's arts district, was constructed in Art Deco style in 1923. A twenty-one-story building historically at full occupancy, it is a site for sophisticated, discerning businesses eager to claim an address in this landmark reminiscent of modernism. On the corner of Spruce and South Broad Streets, one can smell steaks sizzling on pans in Ruth's Chris Steak House, a restaurant on the first floor of the Atlantic Building. The aroma permeates the entrance to the building during the early afternoon and evening hours.

By Jewelers' Row

No margin, no mission, Tine told me emphatically during my visit. Her message was consistent: the nurse–managed model of care *must* be sustainable; nurse practitioners need to *focus, focus, focus*, on reimbursement issues, policy, and politics. The chief executive officer of the Consortium since 1998, Tine grew nurse-managed health centers from 11 to over 250 nationally in a little over ten years. In 2010, the Consortium's budget was over $6.5 million. Tine is good with money; she is also skilled at establishing and sustaining relationships. The Consortium is an affiliate of the Public Health Management Corporation (PHMC), a nonprofit public health institute founded in 1972. Also headquartered on the eighteenth floor of the Atlantic Building, PHMC and its staff work closely with the Consortium on health and human services projects, given their congruent missions and goals. PHMC's administrative structure and tax status facilitate the operation of nursing centers as federally qualified health centers, a designation critical to sustainable care to underserved people. The ties between

PHMC and the Consortium provide a partnership that is wonderfully conducive to taking advantage of opportunistic ventures, which is important to nurse
practitioners. Together, the Consortium and PHMC evaluate health services
provided in the centers, creating an evidence-based portfolio used to match
services to needs, reduce costs, and improve health indices of the patients
they serve. Of critical importance is PHMC's collection of data that compare
nursing center costs to actual patient outcomes. Such analyses lend validity to
arguments advocating for the need for such centers, particularly for vulnerable
populations. PHMC employs nurse practitioners in five nurse-managed sites
located in Philadelphia, all of which are members of the Consortium. PHMC's
administrative infrastructure supports the credentialing of nurse practitioners
as primary care providers with Medicaid, Medicare, and third-party payers.
Jointly, PHMC and the Consortium lobby expertly at state and federal levels to
garner funds and advocate regulatory reform. This intricate, interlaced system
is unified through key leaders.

Passionate about the value of nursing centers—the nursing model of care—
Tine urged nurse practitioners to *hustle more*; to take every opportunity they
can to make professional gains. Leaning forward in her chair in a corner office
bordered by two glass walls, Tine is clearly communicating urgency, a sense
that perhaps the nurse practitioner movement had plateaued in recent years.
Conspiratorial in the way she leans into a conversation, Tine noted that nurse
practitioners are the underdog in the primary care delivery scene and, as such,
must be clear in their strategies to position themselves for reimbursement and
visibility. For example, Tine said, for nurse practitioners to not obtain a U.S.
Department of Justice Drug Enforcement Administration (DEA) number is silly;
to not obtain prescriptive authority is silly. A nurse practitioner can apply for a
number, authorizing her or him to prescribe controlled substances. Controlled
substances such as Percocet—a combination of oxycodone, an opioid analgesic,
and acetaminophen, an analgesic and a fever-reducing medication—and Tylenol with codeine are frequently used to manage pain and require a DEA number to prescribe. Without a DEA number, a nurse practitioner cannot prescribe
what are known as controlled substances in schedules II through IV. Schedule
I drugs are those without current accepted medical use and thus cannot be prescribed; marijuana, heroin, and lysergic acid diethylamide (LSD) are examples
of such drugs. Certain controlled substances are invaluable for management of
commonly occurring symptoms as diverse as acute pain and chronic cough.
Nurse practitioners certified with prescriptive authority by the Pennsylvania
State Board of Nursing may obtain a DEA number from the Office of Diversion
Control, Drug Enforcement Administration.

To practice as an adult nurse practitioner in Pennsylvania, I obtained a license as a Certified Registered Nurse Practitioner (CRNP) from the Pennsylvania Board of Nursing in spring 2008. I also hold license as a CRNP with Prescriptive Authority from the same Board. This license lists my name and the name of my collaborating physician. Without this second license, I am unable to prescribe medications to my patients in Pennsylvania. I also obtained a separate DEA registration number, which must be written on any prescription I write for a controlled dangerous substance. As Tine infers, prescriptive practice, inclusive of a DEA number, is necessary to function as a primary care provider (PCP). *These are not risky behaviors*, states Tine. She also notes that horses taken to water will not necessarily drink. Nurse practitioners, according to Tine, *need more risk-taking and leadership training*; not just care-giver training, if they are to serve as PCPs. Essentially, nurse practitioners must learn to take risks.

One of the nursing centers operated by the Public Health Management Corporation is the Mary Howard Health Center in Philadelphia. Established in 1997, this center is located on the corner of Sansom and Ninth Streets in South Philadelphia, adjacent to Philadelphia's famous Jewelers' Row and the Thomas Jefferson University Hospital emergency department. With many jewelers nestled tightly into brick-lined streets, Jewelers' Row is a stark contrast to the Mary Howard Center. The latter provides care to homeless clients along a continuum of street to shelter to transitional housing to self-sufficiency. I had never taken care of patients in Newark or Camden who were known to be homeless. Though many may have been homeless, their care was provided in the context of a fast-track emergency service or a community center, as I described previously.

The idea of giving primary care to this unique population deeply intrigued me upon joining Temple University in the summer of 2008. Primary care, with the embedded understanding of maintaining a sustained patient-provider relationship over time, seemed impossible to me with homeless patients. However, I soon learned that being homeless did not necessarily mean being transient. After successfully securing my Pennsylvania registered nurse and nurse practitioner licenses, a process that took several months, I requested to work at the Mary Howard Center for a half-day each week. Staffs at both PHMC and the Center were gracious in accepting my request. Allowing a half-day-a-week volunteer provider to give care at the Center created work for PHMC administrators. If eyebrows rose, I didn't see them. I needed to be credentialed as a primary care provider at PHMC and to be accepted as such on health payer panels; additionally, I needed to secure collaborative practice agreements with physicians. The credentialing process was an adventure itself.

Partnering

These credentialing and other processes were time consuming but ultimately successful due to the intervention by Nancy Rothman, EdD, RN, Independence Foundation Endowed Professor of Urban Community Nursing in Temple's Department of Nursing. The Independence Foundation, a private, not-for-profit philanthropic organization serving Philadelphia and its surrounding Pennsylvania counties, supports nurse-managed health care centers. Nancy, a tenured professor within the department I chaired from 2008 to 2012, is funded by both the Independence Foundation and by PHMC. Nancy's role at PHMC is complex, including a primary role for evaluation of evidence-based practice and a secondary, informal role in relationship building and maintenance.

In 1996, Nancy joined Temple University and began working in its previously established wellness and primary care center, the Temple Health Connection, a site located in a public housing community contiguous with Temple's main campus. Funded by a combination of grants and contracts, Temple Health Connection soon became integral to the community it served. Nancy was the cornerstone. Her subtle tenacity and strong, nonthreatening interpersonal skills wove the center into the fabric of the community. She empowered the community to own the center, to plan for services through a strong community advisory group steered gently by her. As sustained external funding sources for primary care became increasingly difficult to secure—and thus the center's primary care services were at risk for continuation—Nancy had looked for partners. She found one in PHMC. In 1997, the Temple Health Connection transferred ownership from Temple University to PHMC, a seamless move with only two ostensible changes: first, a name change to PHMC Health Connection; second, secure funding as one of PHMC's federally qualified health centers—the FQHC status indicating health services reimbursement under the Health Center Consolidation Act 1996. Such secure funding enabled sustainable primary care delivery by nurse practitioners in community-based nursing centers. With increased revenue per patient per visit under the FQHC reimbursement policies, Nancy was now empowered. With primary care services provided under the banner of PHMC Health Connection, Nancy retained the logo "Temple Health Connection" as a vehicle to provide primary health care services, including health education, screening programs, and other services needed by the local community.

Primary care, and primary health care, are two different services. Primary care—the diagnosis and management of acute and chronic illnesses—is provided by nurse practitioners; and primary health care—the management of therapeutic lifestyle choices and health maintenance and illness prevention interventions—is provided by registered nurses. If a patient is diagnosed with hyperlipidemia, or high cholesterol levels, my management most probably will include referral to a dietician for diet management, antihyperlipidemic medications, and referral to a registered nurse for lifestyle management. At the Mary Howard Center, Patty, the registered nurse, would review side effects of medications and when and how to take them, exercise regimens, smoking cessation approaches if applicable, signs of vascular illness (for example, symptoms of a heart attack or a stroke, along with instructions on what to do in these cases), the need for a diet diary, and any aspects of family life or residence that might interrupt the patient's therapeutic plan. Health care reform is dependent on integrated care interventions.

Nancy personally managed the various applications I required to provide primary care provider (PCP) services at the Mary Howard Center. As a nurse practitioner in the fast-track emergency service at University Hospital in Newark, New Jersey, and subsequently in a community site in Camden, I had provided nurse practitioner services, but not as a reimbursable PCP through health insurance payers. Once credentialed at PHMC and approved by health insurance plans, I became a provider whom patients could choose as their PCP. This was different. *Very different.* Up until this point in my career, I provided acute, episodic care requiring the skills of a nurse practitioner, but I had never served as a PCP for continuing care of patients. It was both exciting and frightening. My new role was exciting given that primary care was the nurse practitioner's mantra—the call to arms, the raison d'être, of the movement; the role was frightening because of the attendant responsibility. I felt different, very accountable to my patients and my profession. At age fifty-eight, I had moved from sophisticated volunteerism in Camden to primary care in Philadelphia.

I had kept up with my continuing education readings in primary care, so I felt tentatively comfortable. Since first credentialed as a nurse practitioner in New Jersey, I became an avid consumer of continuing education in primary care. Renewal of licensure as a nurse practitioner in New Jersey and Pennsylvania, as well as renewal of board certification through professional organizations, is contingent upon accrual of continuing education (C.E.) credits. I have a passion for C.E., reading programs in professional journals and online. I find myself excited when my mail includes a professional journal with C.E. in it. I keep up with current medications, new management protocols, and evidence-based research through my c.e. efforts. On planes, on trains, on the beach at Atlantic City, wherever and whenever I have the opportunity, I read c.e. programs. For most programs, I pay a fee to receive my certificate—either in the mail or online. Some programs have no charge, such as those funded by grants. It is remarkably rewarding to receive c.e. certificates. I find that I always have at least one take-away message from each c.e. program—a new drug for migraine headaches, a different way of diagnosing low back pain, treatment regimens for post-traumatic stress disorder, and more.

Here is a confession. In a Temple University administrative retreat in fall 2010, each participant was asked the icebreaker question: What is your favorite book, and why? When it was my turn, I panicked. A book? No. Instead, I told my colleagues about my c.e. habit, a true addiction. I described how I loved to rip open the plastic coverings of my professional journals, anxious to read the table of contents for their monthly c.e. offerings. On the left corner of my desk at home, I pile up my journals, awaiting free moments to luxuriate over the new information or the new approaches to old problems that are housed between these journal covers. My colleagues took a sudden interest in their shoes.

The Mary Howard Center

Before going to the Mary Howard Center for the first time, I had made a trial run. Since I was scheduled on Thursdays from 1 p.m. to 5 p.m., I began my day at the university's health science campus in the morning. Thursday mornings always went fast—program meetings, memo writing, the usual panoply of tasks associated with academic administration. I have always believed that my role as an academic was to ensure high-quality patient care, with students simply as intermediaries in the system. My view is controversial, often shocking to my university colleagues; it hints at a view that education must prepare graduates to contribute to society in meaningful ways, including work preparedness and economic self-sufficiency. Since I focus on patient care, I worry about students' training in critical thinking and diagnostic reasoning—essential tools for safe practice. Educational systems must be superb in order for patient services to be stellar. My outlook explains my passion for scholarly faculty practice. Without a commitment to continued practice as a faculty member, a teacher loses validity among students.

On Thursdays I bring my clinical bag with me to my office, with pride. It contains my cherished tools—a diagnostic set (combined ophthalmoscope/otoscope), a reflex hammer, a tuning fork, a pen light, ear specula, and an odd array of reminders. How to calculate BMI, the stages of hypertension, the how-to's of asthma care, rubrics for diabetes management, the rules for converting from one type of insulin to another, and more.

Stuffed inside my bag is a lab coat with the Temple University Nursing logo and my name embroidered on it. When I originally received my lab coat, one of my cherished administrative nursing colleagues asked if I would now become one of them; the lab coat apparently symbolized something different. She looked sad as she asked the question. Since that interchange, the coat is never visible; rather, it is folded neatly and housed inside my clinical bag. Sigh. My encounter with my valued colleague, while not anticipated, was certainly not a surprise to me. The rift between registered nurses and nurse practitioners is cavernous, almost without bottom.

Giving primary care to my patients takes all my concentration on Thursdays. I have found that if I let myself ruminate over the core issue of oppression among nurses, I become unfocused in my ability to care for my patients. Someday, this rift may close, but only, I believe, if registered nurses receive direct reimbursement for their practice in primary health care delivery. Since our insurance system reimburses for illness care, nurse practitioners receive reimbursement for the care they deliver. This is not true for wellness care; thus, registered nurses are included in administrative bundled service overhead charges. Tine's no-margin, no-mission statement is very relevant to this rift; closing ranks between registered nurses and nurse practitioners will ultimately be more financially beneficial than internally opposing and oppressing each other. Registered nurses must galvanize their power, shifting energy to strategies assuring direct reimbursement for services. Nurse practitioner practice—and nurse practitioners' designation as primary care providers—was a hard-won battle over decades. Registered nurses would do well to pursue this path, preferably with cooperation from nurse practitioners. Our self-oppression makes us easy prey.

My route to the Mary Howard Center is a simple one on Thursdays. I take the Southeastern Pennsylvania Transportation Authority (SEPTA) subway from Temple's health science campus to Center City Philadelphia. I try to get a seat in the first car of the SEPTA train; from this car I can see the interior of the subway tube. The conductor, male or female, usually wears a SEPTA jacket and Dickie pants, and the subway walls are graffiti-laden—an underground community of passengers and conductors that is comfortable and safe. I walk the three-quarter-mile trip from City Hall on Broad Street (Fourteenth Street) to Ninth Street. My walk abounds with contrasts. Initially, I pass loading docks of major buildings, with crowded and narrow streets steamy in summer and bleak in winter. As I get closer to Tenth Street, I feel that I am in the heartland of the Thomas Jefferson University Hospital System. First established in 1825, the system now supports four hospitals and multiple other locations for ambulatory services. I pass stately old buildings rich in history, with people in lab coats or scrub suits scurrying across Sansom, moving between buildings, all imbuing an ambiance of confidence. The buildings I pass speak to history and authority, many with corner plaques dating back to the nineteenth century. The admixture of early American architecture with the functional modernistic buildings of the mid-twentieth century is jarring, almost disrespectful to this historic city.

The Mary Howard Center is located on the corner of Sansom and South Ninth Streets, in a building housing multiple entities. The sign on the thick metal front door states simply: *Mary Howard Health Center.* The door is locked. There is a buzzer to announce your presence and a handle to allow you in.

The center was named after a homeless woman, who, according to Elaine Fox, the vice president for Specialized Health Services at PHMC, was a woman who died falling through the cracks of our health system. Mary Howard, Elaine said, had become the symbol of the struggles of homeless people in Philadelphia. Elaine, with graduate education in sociology, is herself the symbol of advocacy for the homeless. Since 1990, Elaine has managed, coordinated, and advocated for health care access, with emphasis on the homeless population. Whether involved in the Health Care for the Homeless project, the Welfare-to-Work program, the Family Center community, or any of several other programs within her portfolio, Elaine relentlessly pushes her social programs' agendas forward as she consistently meets grant deadlines. I admired Elaine from the first moment I met her: a practical believer, an excellent writer, and a good businesswoman. I see the Mary Howard Center as Elaine's joy.

The Mary Howard Center is in a gray, nondescript building, a stark contrast to the surrounding historic edifices of the Jefferson system. Located on the first floor, with glass walls facing Ninth and Samson Streets, the center is starkly functional, similar to the Community Health Center in Camden. Paper signs taped to the inside of the glass walls announce that N1H1 vaccines are available at the center. One block east is Jewelers' Row.

A Different Definition of Health

When I assumed the position of chair of the nursing department at Temple University in July 2008, I rented a one-room apartment in Center City, Philadelphia. During trips to my grocery store and laundromat, I was stunned by the number of homeless people I saw sleeping on park benches, lying in stairwells of buildings and sheltered by archways, or sleeping over grates on streets under which subways rumbled—with warm air radiating through the grate openings. I have spent my adult life in cities—Newark, Camden, and New York City—but Philadelphia's homeless population seemed disproportionately large by comparison to other urban areas.

Homelessness was acutely visible in Philadelphia. Homelessness—not having a fixed and regular nighttime sleeping residence—is associated with poverty, lack of jobs, and affordable housing. The chronically homeless are those who have been homeless for one or more years or who have experienced four periods of homelessness within three years. Other factors correlate with homelessness—either acute or chronic—and include mental illness, substance abuse, and domestic violence. In 2005, close to fifteen thousand people were served in the city's emergency shelter service. The Mary Howard Health Center, a comprehensive nurse-managed health center for the city's homeless, is funded through a variety of sources—the Philadelphia Department of Health and Human Services, the Independence Foundation, and others. Primary care for homeless residents is also given at two family shelters (Stenton Family Manor located on East Tulpehocken Street and People's Emergency Shelter on Thirty-ninth Street, both in Philadelphia) and two other nurse-managed health centers (Rising Sun on the corner of Adams Street and Rising Sun Avenue in North Philadelphia and the PHMC Health Connection at Eleventh Street and Berks Street adjacent to Temple University's main campus). In 2010, the Care Clinic on Callowhill Street was added as a site for primary care, with a special history of treating persons with HIV/AIDS. Collectively, these sites are a coordinated safety net for homeless individuals and their families in the city of Philadelphia. In 2010, eleven hundred homeless residents were serviced by this network of primary care, behavioral health, and social services programs linked by Philadelphia's Health Care for the Homeless (HCH) Program and administered by PHMC.

I had never before worked exclusively with homeless patients. As a nurse practitioner in the fast-track service of University Hospital's emergency department, I had, of course, encountered homeless patients. My focus there was acute episodic care, not primary care; and, as a relatively new practitioner at that time, I was so overwhelmingly concerned about getting patients' histories, physical examination findings, and diagnoses correct that homelessness was not on my radar screen. I recall one patient telling me that he usually lived in a van with a friend, and another who called Newark's Branch Brook Park his home. I knew homelessness then, but it was a two-dimensional concept to me at that time. And, while I knew intellectually that discharge planning is important, I also appreciated that it seemed somewhat futile for such patients. Giving such patients follow-up appointments to medical clinics, or handing them prescriptions to fill for generic drugs, were the correct actions to take; however, even then I doubted that the appointments would be kept or the prescriptions filled. A system did not exist for managing such complex patients.

I was oriented on my first day at the center. There were three full-time adult nurse practitioners, one psychiatric/mental health nurse practitioner, one part-time adult nurse practitioner, one registered nurse, two medical assistants, one social worker, one referral staff member, one appointment clerk, and a part-time dietitian. One-stop shopping. I was most impressed with the full-time social worker, who is especially important for these clients and their complex housing, social, and welfare needs. I immediately sensed a community, a community of all women. I was reminded of Carol Gilligan's writing—*In a Different Voice: Psychological Theory and Women's Development* (1982)—with its emphasis on women's sense of connectivity giving rise to a sense of responsibility for one another. This sense was clearly present and pervasive. Also present was a community of nurse practitioners—primary care providers—who relied on each other for help, consultation with differential diagnoses, sharing interesting laboratory results, and other patient concerns. Without a physician present, it was a different health delivery world. It was a horizontal system, with the concept of homelessness ever present as a unifying theme, and felt quite liberating since my first moment in the center. As I shadowed one adult nurse practitioner on my first day, I began to appreciate the relationships that existed. My mentor was revered for her clinical acumen and broad experiences in primary care, as well as for her gentleness. The psychiatric/mental health nurse practitioner was the community's glue, defusing tension and helping the group to stay on course, to be practical in what could, and couldn't, be accomplished on any one day. I immediately felt welcomed, the token academic nurse practitioner who still wanted to retain a life in practice. They were patient with me, with my slowness and repetitive questions regarding the electronic medical record.

My first patient was a middle-aged African American male with complaints of vomiting bright red blood on and off for the past three days. He was nauseous. His skin was pale, his abdomen distended, and his arms and legs were thin, with multiple ecchymotic and bruised areas. His history was straightforward: twenty- to thirty-year history of extensive alcohol use interspersed with participation in several substance abuse treatment programs. *I couldn't do it. I always went back*, he said. My years in medical intensive care had exposed me to alcoholic cirrhosis, gastroesophageal varices, and gastrointestinal bleeding. He was uninsured. Fearing major GI bleeding, I referred him to a local emergency department for diagnostics and management. The registered nurse, Miss Pat, called ahead to local hospitals and eventually escorted him to Pennsylvania Hospital, just a few blocks south of the center on Spruce Street. I called ahead and spoke with the charge nurse in the emergency department, who seemed curious as to why I felt the need to call in the first place.

This patient, a walk-in, did not return to the center, and I did not receive any follow-up information regarding him. From my days in emergency rooms, I was accustomed to patients being treated and never seen again. Most were discharged, with a few admitted to the hospital. I came to appreciate, however, that in primary care practice, it is disconcerting to have patients simply disappear. I had come to expect follow-up with patients, to develop relationships, to counsel patients on more than simply the management of disease. Over time in primary care, I incorporated a more complex definition of health in my practice—was the patient satisfied with his achievements in education? Did he want more training and a better income? Was he satisfied with social security disability income or welfare income? Did he want to improve his interpersonal communication skills, his partnership relationship? To lose patients to follow-up care is disturbing.

For the first few months at the center I saw only walk-in patients, including those who were regular patients without scheduled appointments but who were experiencing acute illnesses, or patients who were new to the center. Dealing with walk-ins was more similar than dissimilar to managing fast-track emergency department patients. They presented with acute needs, whether physical, mental, or dental. Some new patients included those staying at Coleman Hall, an education and treatment center on D Street in North Philadelphia. Many residents at Coleman Hall include those referred through the state's Department of Corrections, the Pennsylvania Board of Probation and Parole, or the Bucks County Department of Corrections. Founded in 2001, Coleman Hall provides reentry treatment services aimed at reducing recidivism.

Residents at Coleman Hall, as well as others, often request the completion of a form termed the Employability Assessment Form (EAF). The EAF, distributed by the Pennsylvania Department of Public Welfare, requires a provider to attest to a patient's eligibility for medical assistance benefits on the basis of a medical evaluation by a physician or a certified registered nurse practitioner. If the patient is evaluated as being temporarily or permanently disabled, then he or she will be reviewed for medical assistance benefits. The definition of disabled is left to the judgment of the provider conducting the examination.

Initially, I found this form to be challenging. How is disability operationally defined? Throughout my clinical career, my goal has been to assist people to meet their goals and enjoy a quality of life based on their strengths, often irrespective of disabilities. Could not all physically capable people be able to engage in some type of meaningful work? My understandings of this broad construct—disability—deepened as I dealt with the patients at this center. Health, clearly, is much more than the absence of physical disease. It is also more than the absence of mental illness, or psychiatric labels. Maintenance of health requires organizational skill, daily stamina, the executive ability to prioritize based on long-term goals and objectives. One must learn to get on a bus at a specific time, to set an alarm clock, to reject temptation to nap or to hang around with unemployed friends, to refrain from old drug and/or alcohol habits, to become increasingly self-disciplined. Newly released prisoners without work skills, support networks, past employment successes, organizational executive abilities, hardiness and self-reliance—even in the absence of physical or mental disease—are disabled. My graduate student education framed my appreciation for complexity, helping me to recognize the multidimensionality of concepts embedded in any one construct. Disability is a complex construct, with concepts of poverty, illness, homelessness, and more incorporated within it. Homeless patients sleeping at night within shelters or other facilities also seek completion of the EAF. I found myself estimating how long a person can be homeless before he or she can be termed temporarily disabled.

To understand more deeply the context of disability in my homeless patients, I sought help from my colleague in social work, a person I had known previously from the Hispanic Family Center of Southern New Jersey in Camden. She, and the psychiatric/mental health nurse practitioner, deepened my understanding of the conceptual links tying homelessness and disability together—two sides of a single, complex phenomenon. Giving a homeless patient time—checking off temporary disability for six months—to acquire the skills needed to find, and retain, a job and affordable housing is an intervention equal to, or better then, a prescription for a medication or therapy. Some simply need time to obtain stamina, skills, and a fresh orientation to living. My repertoire was expanding. Completing the EAF takes professional maturity, sensitivity to patients' contexts and needs, and required time from me.

At the Mary Howard Health Center, I began to see patients who returned to me for continuing primary care. I was very pleased and very vigilant. Providing continuing primary care is radically different from giving acute episodic care. In continuing care, patients come back to you. They tell you how the plan of care did or didn't work, given their lifestyles. I facilitate patients' planning their care, but I cannot single-handedly dictate a plan of care. Clearly, plans for continuing care need to evolve from patients, with guidance from the nurse practitioner.

One of my first routine continuing-care patients was a fifty-eight-year-old African American male with hypertension, Bill. Bill had been homeless for more than twenty years; he claimed one particular bench in Rittenhouse Square Park as his. He knew the names of the morning joggers. Most of them, he said, worked in hospitals. At night he slept in a shelter. During the day he walked around Center City. He thought of himself as a helper to other homeless people, giving them information on shelters and food pantries. He had Stage 2 hypertension, a type requiring two or more medications to control. Following accepted recommendations from evidence-based practice, I offered him a thiazide diuretic and a calcium channel blocker, both to be taken once daily in the morning. He took the drug samples, saying that he would try to remember to take them. Living in a shelter is difficult, and frequently, he reported, you lose your medicines or they get stolen. When he returned for a follow-up visit a few weeks later, his blood pressure had only inched minimally in the right direction. When asked if he routinely took his two medications, he said no, it was just too hard to take both. The diuretic had made his life miserable. He couldn't find public bathrooms fast enough when the urge to urinate hit him; his quality of life was deteriorating, even if his headaches and occasional nosebleeds were getting less frequent. *What do you want to do?* I asked. He would take two pills, *just not a water pill, please, not a water pill.* We settled on two drugs, one considered very effective in African Americans, plus a commonly prescribed second medication. I was learning to negotiate and compromise—valuable skills in patient-focused care.

As I negotiated plans of care, I wondered what risks I was taking. One learns fast in health care that you are judged by your peers as to the safety and appropriateness of your plan of care. Who are my peers? Certainly only other providers who managed homeless patients. In a court, however, it may be different: my peers would be other adult nurse practitioners. Would an adult nurse practitioner practicing in an ambulatory practice in an affluent suburban community be my peer? If yes, would he or she typically negotiate with patients regarding what type of antihypertensive they were willing to take? Still, I would rather work with these patients in this setting than engage in a standard, template practice based on a medical model in a physician's office. I write a prescription—enroll in a community college and obtain advice from an academic counselor—as a treatment, reflecting my broad definition of health that might alarm my peers. What, I can hear the jury cry, has *that* to do with health care?

Shortly thereafter I met John, a fifty-seven-year-old African American male who had broken his right ankle in a fall near the Hospital of the University of Pennsylvania (HUP). He had been homeless for several years, occasionally sleeping at his daughter's home—*until she can't stand me anymore*—or, more frequently at a shelter. He had Keystone Mercy Medicaid health insurance. When he was injured, he was taken to HUP's emergency department. He was taught RICE treatment—rest, ice, compression ace bandages, and elevation of his leg above the level of his heart. At HUP, he had also been given Percocet for pain, a medication combining oxycodone—a narcotic—with acetaminophen, an analgesic and fever-relieving medication, to be taken as needed every six hours. His blood pressure was so elevated that the orthopedic surgeon on consult requested that he return to the Mary Howard Center to control his hypertension prior to surgical intervention. I treated him according to textbook protocol—two medications and follow-up visits weekly. His blood pressure did not decrease with the anti-hypertension regimen. I added clonidine, a medication often used in emergency situations to decrease dangerously high blood pressure. When he took one 0.2 mg tablet of clonidine during one visit to the center, his blood pressure decreased within an hour to a Stage 1 reading. He was then convinced to take the clonidine, but only one of the other two drugs. We compromised on clonidine and the calcium channel blocking drug, nifedipine.

Over several weeks, John was evaluated by the HUP orthopedic surgeon while I managed his primary care needs at the center. He continuously complained of pain. At one visit, he told me that his Percocets had been stolen and that he needed a refill. I did not give him another prescription, given that the common practice at the center was to refuse a refill before the first prescription was complete, particularly for patients such as John with a substance abuse history. Shortly thereafter, he developed osteomyelitis in his ankle and his surgeon prescribed long-term antibiotics prior to reviewing him for any surgical intervention. The surgeon also prescribed Percocet for pain. When John returned to me for primary care, he was still taking his antibiotic, clonidine, and nifedipine. He had lost weight—ten pounds. While he was taking antibiotics, his daughter allowed him to stay with her. His blood pressure was under control.

He collapsed in the chair in my little examination room, propping his crutches against the wall and taking his protective boot off his right ankle. He said he was in pain. I believed him. He had been emergency room hopping for pain medication for the past week, going to Jefferson University Hospital and HUP. He had been given pain medications in both hospitals, as is common practice. How do you provide pain management for patients with histories of drug addiction? I conferred with the nurse practitioner following him at HUP to gain her perspective on management of John's pain. His osteomyelitis was severe, requiring open incision and drainage through a three-inch surgical incision along the dorsum of his right foot, along with postoperative intravenous antibiotics. I wrote a prescription for basic laboratory diagnostics—blood chemistries, liver panel, and lipid profile—and then a prescription for Percocet for pain. I gave him enough tablets for pain control for three weeks, at the end of which time he would return for evaluation of his blood pressure, pain, osteomyelitis, and fracture, with the intent of comanaging him with his HUP orthopedic surgeon.

As I wrote my DEA number on the prescription for John and called in my National Provider Identifier number—a unique identification number for each covered health care provider that is used in administrative and financial transactions adapted under the Health Insurance Portability and Accountability Act—to the pharmacist, I was reminded of the responsibilities inherent in primary care. Relationships with patients take trust—and risk-taking. I thought of John frequently over the weeks that I managed his primary care needs and his pain. I did not hesitate to write prescriptions for Endocet—the generic form of Percocet that he preferred—but I also collected urine samples for drug screens (to determine if he was taking the Endocet or diverting the pills to others) and spoke with him about referrals to a pain management group. My internal heuristic for practice emphasized balance between trust and evidence. What, a jury of my peers might wonder, has *that* to do with health care?

The Shot Nurse?

One Thursday afternoon at the Mary Howard Center, as I escorted a patient to the main office to schedule his follow-up visit, two staff members in the triage area were helping a young man into a chair. Twenty-four years old, disheveled in appearance and irritable in behavior, this patient—Daryl—was extremely hypoglycemic. His blood glucose was 45 mg, below the normal range of 80 mg to 120 mg. One of the medical assistants gave him a glass of orange juice; the other gave him a granola bar. He seemed to rally quickly. Once he stabilized and his vital signs, weight, height, BMI, chief complaint, family history, and social history were documented in the triage area, he was brought back to me as a walk-in. He was quiet, head down, fingers fidgeting with his paperwork held tightly in his hand. He needed to have a physical examination documented so that his Employability Assessment Form could be returned to the Pennsylvania Department of Public Welfare. Was he disabled? Living in a shelter at night, he walked around the city most of the day, seeing if anyone needed him to do odd

jobs. He was a vague historian. Was he a reliable narrator? I doubted the verac-
ity of his story. Without doubt, however, he was diabetic. He said he had been
diabetic since he was nine years old, almost fifteen years. He had taken insulin
injections for years, once in the morning and once in the evening—a combination of fast-acting insulin with short-acting insulin. His physical examination
was unremarkable, barring his underweight status and general appearance of
poor nutrition and poor hygiene. His fidgety behaviors and anxious mood were
noteworthy, as were his expressions of feeling sad most of the time. I completed his form, evaluating him as temporarily disabled for six months. On the
encounter form that I returned to the office manager, I checked diabetes mellitus Type 1, underweight/malnutrition, and anxiety as diagnoses. I wrote him
prescriptions for NPH insulin and insulin syringes, and I referred him to the
psychiatric/mental health nurse practitioner for evaluation. I also referred him
to the registered nurse for diabetic education. Since he was uninsured, I did
not write a prescription for laboratory work, commonly collected to confirm
the diagnosis of diabetes. For the prescriptions for the insulin and syringes, I
sent him to a local pharmacy that cooperates with the center; on the prescription I indicated that the center would pay for the prescriptions. Again, risk. I
was treating diabetes without confirmation of serum glucose or glycosylated
hemoglobin; my only data were his history and his current glucose value by
fingerstick.

   On the encounter form used for billing purposes as well as documentation of referrals and next appointments, I checked off three diagnoses for this
patient. Each of these diagnoses had a corresponding International Classification of Diseases (ICD) code. The ICD codes provide information regarding financial charges established for any particular diagnosis. These codes have been
approved by the four organizations that compose the cooperating parties for the
codes—the American Hospital Association, the American Health Information
Management Association, the Centers for Medicare and Medicaid Services, and
the National Center for Health Statistics. My patient's codes included diabetes mellitus Type 1 uncontrolled (250.01), underweight (783.22), and anxiety
unspecified (300.00). Without health insurance, I had made the diagnosis of
diabetes presumptively. Normally, a diagnosis of diabetes is made on the basis
of blood work, either a fasting blood glucose test or an oral glucose tolerance
test. A valuable test to determine the average plasma glucose concentration
over time is the simple glycosylated hemoglobin—or HbA1c—test, which can
be used to monitor improvement in a diabetic patient over time. As I thought
about this patient later, wondering if he would return for follow-up management once he received his health insurance card, I realized that I could have

ordered an HbA1c while he was in the center. The center would have paid for this test, given his lack of insurance at the time, but the key was in patient management. It would have been a simple, relatively inexpensive way to determine his general diabetes state. Even without all of the data on hand from which to make a diagnosis or determine a plan of care, I still had to act.

I was very comfortable in referring this diabetic patient to the registered nurse for diabetes education. Primary care providers diagnose and manage deviations from wellness, ordering diagnostic tests and procedures, referring to specialists, and prescribing medications, devices, and other therapies such as physical therapy and occupational therapy. Registered nurses provide patient education, the key link between disease management and health maintenance.

The legislative background that set the stage for such collaboration is relatively recent. In 2007, Pennsylvania's governor Edward Rendell initiated legislation called Prescription for Pennsylvania, an effort to address the quality of care, health promotion, and cost containment. A critical component in this legislation was the mandate to employ nurse practitioners as primary care providers. In 2009, the Mary Howard Center's nurse practitioners managed thousands of visits, receiving reimbursement as staff of a federally qualified health center. By enabling nurse practitioners to serve as PCPs, more patients are served. Acute episodic illnesses are treated; chronic illnesses are managed. I learned quickly at the center that time is an important variable in the overall management of patients, either for acute or chronic illness management. With patients lining up like jets on a runway at John F. Kennedy Airport in New York City, I knew to focus on accurately diagnosing and outlining a management plan in my PCP role, and I needed to do so as quickly as possible. Time is not on the side of a PCP with regard to thoroughly educating patients either about their medications or recommended therapeutic lifestyle changes. Once diagnosed correctly and with a mutually-agreed-upon management regimen, patients need education in order to manage their illness, initiate lifestyle changes, prevent costly and time-consuming complications, and generally improve their overall quality of life—all the while incorporating chronic illness into their lifestyles and daily patterns.

It was at the Mary Howard Center, thirty-seven years after becoming a registered nurse, that I fully realized the critical role of the registered nurse in primary health care. The health indices of our patients will not radically shift in a positive direction if health education is not provided. Pat, the registered nurse at the Mary Howard Center, became my metaphor for primary health care delivery by registered nurses. For Daryl to understand his disease and to manage his life—food, medications, exercise—and to prevent complications of diabetes, he must return to be taught how to inject his insulin, plan meals and get tips on calorie-counting, learn how to use the glucometer, be given time to ask questions, and much more. He would need to thoroughly understand the signs and symptoms of the most common complications of diabetes, including hypoglycemia, hyperglycemia, infection, neuropathy, visual problems, and side effects of medications. He would need to know why it is important to get the HbA1c test every few months. He must be in charge—in charge of his wellness, his daily diabetes management, and his lifestyle choices.

I am fully aware that I cannot provide this thorough education, given the realities of primary care time constraints. No margin, no mission. But Pat can. The Pennsylvania Code Title 49, Professional and Vocational Standards, defines the practice of professional nursing capaciously as "diagnosing and treating human responses to actual or potential health problems through such services as case findings, health teaching, health counseling, provision of care supportive to or restorative of life and well-being, and executive medical regimens as prescribed by a licensed physician or dentist." Working as an intradisciplinary team, registered nurses and nurse practitioners can both improve access to primary care as well as increase patient outcomes through education. I managed patients' primary care and Pat promoted healthy lifestyle choices and intense education—teamwork.

"Incident to" Billing

In May 2007, the Pennsylvania Chronic Care Management, Reimbursement, and Cost Reduction Commission was established. The commission's strategic plan, published in February 2008, called for a radical shift in focus, from an acute hospitalist perspective to the control of chronic disease in context. It also called for reimbursement for effective control of chronic conditions, care coordination, and office systems that prevent hospitalizations and emergency department visits. Public Health Management Corporation (PHMC) and the staff at the Mary Howard Center quickly seized this opportunity. A new clinical protocol entitled *Protocol for Registered Nurses to See Newly Diagnosed or Unstable Patients with Chronic Illnesses* became effective in March 2010, and called for registered nurses to be reimbursed for services delivered to newly diagnosed or unstable patients by direction of the certified registered nurse practitioner. The nurse's care would then be provided incident to the nurse practitioner. On the encounter form, the visit to the RN is determined to be a Level I visit—a Current Procedural Terminology (CPT) encounter code 99211. The CPT encounter code 99211 is applied to the evaluation and management of a patient that may not require the presence of a primary care provider. Reporting RN visits incident to the nurse practitioner benefit both the patient and the practice. The patient receives the education vitally needed and the practice—the Mary Howard Center—receives payment for this visit. As noted by a physician assistant, Emily Hill, in "Understanding When to Use 99211: Using CPT Code 99211 Can Boost Your Practice's Revenue and Improve Documentation" (*Family Practice Management,* 2004), the CPT code 99211 level I can boost your practice's revenue and improve documentation. Hill noted that the majority of providers fail to capture 99211 charges; she advised primary care providers to recall that all services create costs, noting that the 99211 are easy revenue. Reporting all costs to the center will also provide data for evidence-based practice; documenting outcomes of patients taught therapeutic lifestyle changes by nurses validate these interventions and provide a database for further research.

In January 2011, I received a letter from Keystone Mercy Health Plan that welcomed me to the Keystone Mercy network—I was successfully credentialed as a nurse practitioner. Credentialed as a primary care provider, I had accomplished a major career goal, almost forty years in planning. With my provider number in hand, patients at the Mary Howard Health Center could now choose me as their primary care provider, or PCP. After decades of seeking recognition to bill for services independently, I found the simple three-paragraph form letter in my hand almost anticlimactic. I filed my letter. I now knew the responsibility involved in the acronym *PCP.*

Managing medical care for people with low incomes who meet state criteria for Medicaid benefits began in 1965 with Public Law 89–97: Social Security Act Amendments of 1965, Title XIX, the law that created both the Medicare and Medicaid programs. By 2011, Medicaid had become the third-largest source of health insurance in the country, after employer-based plans and Medicare. Medicaid, the country's safety net program, protects vulnerable populations and designated eligibility groups, including low-income women, children, the elderly, and those with disabilities. In 1995, New Jersey's Medicaid program shifted their insured clients from traditional fee-for-service programs into managed care programs; thus, Medicaid recipients enrolled in Health Maintenance Organizations (HMOs), choosing their PCPs from among such organizations' lists of approved providers. With a shift to a medical home—through the PCP—and a comprehensive array of prevention services, the inappropriate delivery of primary care in expensive hospital emergency departments was supposed to slow down, if not cease altogether.

Similarly, by 2007, 72 percent of Medicaid recipients in Pennsylvania had been enrolled in an HMO, as is reported in their online reports. In Pennsylvania, the Medicaid program is commonly called Medical Assistance, a program administered by the Department of Public Welfare. Mandatory managed care for all Medical Assistance recipients in Pennsylvania occurred by 2001. The majority of federal money provided to states through the Medicaid program that supports Community Health Centers (CHCs) is channeled into sites designated as Federally Qualified Health Centers (FQHCs). The FQHC program, established in 1989 by the U.S. Congress, supports care through either a prospective payment system (PPS) that provides a per visit payment rate for each FQHC in advance, or an approved alternate payment system such as the retention of a cost-based reimbursement system. FQHCs allow billable encounters by nurse practitioners and physician assistants that would be covered if furnished by a physician, provided that the nurse practitioner or physician assistant is legally permitted to perform the services by the State in which they are performed, as described in the Code of Federal Regulations Title 42: Public Health. Once a medical record patient encounter is opened by a provider, payment will relate to the services provided by that provider. Payment for services rendered by FQHCs is increased through supplemental payments—wraparound payments—that enhance services provided, including, for example, primary prevention services such as pneumococcal and influenza vaccines. Wrap-around payments to the Mary Howard Health Center, for example, provide sustainable revenue to provide comprehensive medical and social services to complex patients.

Once credentialed as a PCP by Keystone Mercy Health Plan, I determined to understand how my own services are billed at Mary Howard. As nurse practitioners evolved in their practice, a key agenda item was independent billing for health services provided. Initially, nurse practitioners billed under the incident to option of Medicare; that is, their services were billed under the collaborating physician's provider number, as long as services were provided in the physician's practice site and the nurse practitioner was directly supervised by the physician. Revenue would go to the physician, with nurse practitioners as salaried professional staff. Over time, nurse practitioners have achieved independent billing for their services, at 85 percent of the physician fee schedule for the same service. As physician practices face increasing costs and decreasing reimbursements, the employment of nurse practitioners becomes increasingly attractive to them. As observed by Michael Lowe in May 2008, "Incident-to billing presents one of the last remaining opportunities for them [physicians] to multiply their services and increase their income without having to work harder" (*Orlando Medical News*, May 2008).

Such practice leaves room for fraud. Providers and institutions that falsely bill for services that violate billing regulations are charged with fraud by

Medicare and Medicaid. In 1996, public records indicate that the Clinical Practices of the University of Pennsylvania had to pay the federal government more than $30 million for errors, including the billing of Medicare for the alleged services of attending physicians when the services were actually performed by resident physicians. Records also show that at the University of Medicine and Dentistry of New Jersey, a $2 million settlement was paid to the government in 2009 to settle allegations under the False Claims Act that it double billed Medicaid by nearly $5 million.

As Tine Hansen-Turton, CEO of the National Nursing Centers Consortium and vice president of Public Health Management Corporation, had told me early in my career at Temple University: *No Margin, No Mission.*

Practice to Education

As my perspective broadened at the Mary Howard Center with patients such as Daryl, I rolled my epiphanies over to the Temple nursing curriculum. Temple University academic nursing has a long history, having been established in 1893 by the institution's founder, Pastor Russell Conwell. As with Newark City Hospital School of Nursing (the precursor to the School of Nursing at the University of Medicine and Dentistry of New Jersey), which had been established during that same period, the orientation to health care had a modern-era, hospitalist focus on acute illness care—the management of disease by physicians assisted by registered nurses. Even with Harvard University widely expanding its degree offerings in the early twentieth century, nursing focused on acute care and apprenticeship training.

It was no surprise to me that Temple's undergraduate Bachelor of Science in Nursing (BSN) program in 2008 had a course entitled "Medical-Surgical Nursing." That was a pivotal year for change. Barack Obama was elected president of the United States, and in March 2010 he signed Public Law 111–148—Patient Protection and Affordable Care Act.

This law marked steps toward a paradigm shift—from the modern era hospital disease management focus to the postmodern, global-era focus on access and health care—that rivets attention on the patient rather than the provider, to the care delivered rather than to the provider delivering it, driving down services to the least costly provider. That same month—March 2010—Temple's nursing faculty endorsed new organizing constructs through which the curricula would shift from hospitalist to primary health care. These constructs—professional self-regulations, health promotion, global health, disease prevention, integrated care services, ethical practice, evidence-based practice, and leadership—emanated from tenets outlined by the Declaration of Alma-Ata at the International Conference on Primary Care sponsored by the World Health Organization in 1978. Alignment began in 2010 among a number of variables, not the least of which were the underlying philosophical beliefs of the very faculty responsible for graduating nurse providers with a new outlook and skills; here was an outlook consistent with their scope of practice—diagnosis and treatment of human responses to actual or potential health problems. As the faculty became engaged in—and excited about—our revolution to shift students' attention to primary care, I became more confident.

Since my early experiences as an academic administrator at UMDNJ, I have felt an urgency to do away with the standard nursing curriculum, with its emulation of medicine's specialties and its unacknowledged desire to meet the demands of hospital administrators. In 1893, when the American Society of Superintendents of Training Schools for Nurses—the forerunner of the National League for Nursing—was established, the profession mandated the standardization of a uniform curriculum. Ever since, nursing educators have ceaselessly demanded compliance to a standard curriculum. And, given nursing's historic focus on physicians rather than patients, nursing curricula generally continue to be framed around medicine's big five clinical services—medicine, surgery, pediatrics, obstetrics, and psychiatry. While other content in community health, public health, and management has been incorporated incrementally since the mid-twentieth century, nurse educators are unconsciously drawn back to the big five, like lemmings to the sea. Compliance and obedience to the standard curriculum was rewarded with unquestioned accreditation of programs, with deviance simply not tolerated.

In the late 1980s, I joined the American Association of Colleges of Nursing on behalf of UMDNJ. Established in 1969, the AACN has aimed to promote educational standards and provide advocacy for policies and legislation regarding higher education initiatives in nursing. At one annual conference, a debate ensued about the challenges of offering nursing education within academic health science universities. The issue—that the needs of academic medicine could potentially overwhelm or overshadow those of academic nursing—resulted in lively conversation. My interpretation of this conversation was simple. Academic health science centers, with the hospital as the central hub of activity, focus on illness, medical care, and the care delivered by others (nurses and allied health providers) in the overall service of managing medical diagnoses.

I returned home to my UMDNJ campus with a goal: to shift our curricular focus from illness to health, from provider to patient. It seemed obvious to me that we needed to radically crank into another gear if we were to focus our education on wellness, on keeping people out of hospitals. It seemed sensible, simple. I convened faculty, urged a move to lifestyle management, even suggested new courses (e.g., "Healthy Lifestyles") to replace traditional courses (e.g., "Acute Adult Medical-Surgical Nursing"). They listened to me, but continued the established programs without change.

Quite a failure.

A few years later, when President Bill Clinton advocated for an expanded role of nurses in a reforming health system, I had hoped that the nursing faculty could provide care to students at UMDNJ. The faculty was irate, however, refusing to be the *shot nurses* in the Student Health Center. My notion that the registered nurse license gave faculty opportunities to educate students on healthy lifestyles, safe sexual practices, and other topics did not attract volunteers to the center. I had the sense that such efforts were deemed lowly, not requiring the services of an educated person. One person told me *I didn't get my doctorate to do that!* This effort failed, as did national health care reform at that time. My steamrolling approach at UMDNJ was not endearing.

The Temple faculty, over time, endorsed the concept of curricular reform and themselves began the process of revising courses in 2010. I felt a sense of closure. In the intervening period between the Clinton and Obama administrations, the poor lifestyle choices of many Americans had gained national attention, particularly evident in obesity statistics. Many interacting factors, not the least of which was an increasing acceptability of lifestyle management as a real intervention (in fact, a very fashionable intervention!), had converged in 2010 to do the unthinkable—revise the standardized nursing curriculum. Lunatic fringe or avant garde? Would our revised curriculum open up new approaches to our science, as Thomas Kuhn's *The Structure of Scientific Revolutions* would suggest? Paradigms shift when our explanations no longer capture events. If the aphorism "no margin, no mission" is true, then educating for lifestyle management as intervention makes sense. At this, the jury of my peers would knowingly nod.

A Different Kind of Care

On my way to the Mary Howard Health Center one warm, sunny afternoon in September without a hint of humidity, I felt unusually at peace. It was a day with a mild, cool breeze and a sun that created incredibly sharp shadows on city sidewalks. People lingered on the sidewalks, getting their lunches from street vendors lined up on Ninth Street, outside the U.S. Post Office, a five-story building of massive masonry built in 1884 with porticoed granite columns and an interior first floor housing forty-two service windows, not all of which are currently in use. There were many places to lean against comfortably and enjoy an outside lunch, a hot cup of afternoon coffee. Just to see the interior of this grand building, I stood on line for twenty minutes to purchase a book of stamps. I love Philadelphia, the magnificently bold buildings, speaking to an era of grandiosity, announcing our country's entrance onto the international scene. One feels it is still a young country, but a historic city, admixed with ATM machines in magnificent old edifices. The day before I had met with Dr. Donald Parks, one of the two physicians with whom I have collaborative practice agreements required by Pennsylvania's State Board of Nursing to engage in primary care practice. My agreement with Dr. Parks provides me with the privilege of prescriptive authority, an essential part of primary care.

I had met Dr. Parks earlier, but not to speak with individually. He and I had provided comments in spring 2010, when the Institute of Medicine, in collaboration with the Robert Wood Johnson Foundation, conducted an on-site visit to the Temple Health Connection as a part of its 2011 report *The Future of Nursing: Leading Change, Advancing Health.* A panel of several committee members was hosted by Temple's Nancy Rothman and others who were on-site at the community health center that was located in public housing adjacent to the university's main campus.

Dr. Parks's primary care practice with nurse practitioners extended his services in the North Philadelphia area he served. He cared for many patients with multiple health problems; he saw nurse practitioners as helping him provide access to these patients. When grilled about any disadvantages of practicing collaboratively with nurse practitioners, Dr. Parks was silent. No, he saw no disadvantages. I visited with him a few months later, with an interview schedule in hand. He graciously gave an hour on a Wednesday, his day to catch up with office work. His office, located on North Broad Street in an old home with twenty-six rooms built in 1880, reflects his demeanor and personality. Brownstone on the outside with high tin ceilings on the inside—commonplace in the late nineteenth century, the building has been only minimally retrofitted to serve as a medical office. The waiting room, its walls lined with locked, glass-encased bookshelves housing hundreds of unopened toys of black heroes, heroines, Barbie dolls, GI Joes, and others, has chairs arranged along the walls' perimeters. These toys, gifts from patients and others, have accumulated over the years. The central office area, with several desks and staff members looking very much in charge of their functions, is also expansive, with desks clearly identified by the pictures and other personal effects of the individuals occupying those spaces. Dr. Parks's office, with chairs surrounding his large desk, is equally individualistic and inviting. A busy place. Workers move from the central office area through

Dr. Parks's office, waving their hands in a gesture of hello to the physician responsible for this island of activity. Nods of heads, smiles. Warmth uncommon for an ambulatory medical practice.

Do you want a copy of my CV? Dr. Parks asked. He gave me his CV and business cards, one for his practice site and one for his Temple University title— Assistant Dean, Minority Affairs, and Director, Center for Minority Health Studies. Temple Nursing's graduate program, he applauded, did a good job at selecting students for admission to its nurse practitioner program. Temple students, he added, fit the community. Dr. Parks charmed me. Our graduate program is relatively small in numbers, a fact that I have worried about. I hope our numbers will increase. While it is nice to graduate great practitioners, administrators internal to the college frown on our selective enrollments. Taking notes, I focused on Dr. Parks's comments. We agreed—a lot of graduates are good, but good graduates are best. We discussed our program in North Philadelphia and our mission to prepare primary care providers for urban populations, our niche market. We attract local residents to our programs, the majority of whom remain in the area after graduation. My confidence increased.

Confident in my academic knowledge of primary care, but aware of my slowness in a busy practice setting and my relative ineptness in mastering the electronic medical record, I usually approach each Thursday afternoon with a combination of excitement and nervousness. As I entered the center this particular September afternoon, however, I was relaxed, a nice feeling. My hour with Dr. Parks had incidental outcomes, far beyond gathering the data I had wished to obtain. Dr. Parks, in addition to serving as a collaborative practice physician, also served as a preceptor for graduate nurse practitioner students. When I asked him how we could improve our program, he had smiled and asked me to give the students more time in a busy office; they need time to learn the flow of patient care in ambulatory practice. They need to learn how to focus on the *single main issue* that patients present with. Nurses, Dr. Parks said, worked under a different model of care—the nursing model. In primary care, they need to transition to a different model because now they are not giving nursing care. As Tine Hansen-Turton had said, nurse practitioners need to *focus, focus, and focus again.* Tine had been advocating for a focus on policy and politics; Dr. Parks, a busy primary care provider, urged nurse practitioners to focus on chief complaints, rather than total health—*they don't need to do a million-dollar workup*, he said, smiling. Yes, focus. I could learn to focus.

My first patient that afternoon was Sam, a forty-seven-year-old man, lean and athletic in build, with a big grin and gaps in his upper front teeth. Both knees were wrapped in Ace bandages that had long ago lost their elasticity, marked with blood and dirt stains. Limping, Sam made his way through the makeshift hallways of the center, which was now undergoing expansion. With grant funds awarded through the American Recovery and Reinvestment Act of 2009, the Public Health Management Corporation began to implement an expansion project to the Mary Howard Health Center in early 2010 that would increase patient examination rooms from five to ten. As my patient navigated through the narrow hallway draped with plastic barriers and temporarily cramped spaces, I listened to his story of having been shot in both knees one weekend earlier. *I was in the wrong place at the wrong time.* One bullet entered his right anterior thigh above his knee, exited posterior, and then entered his left knee, exiting without entering bone. He had been treated at Temple University Hospital's emergency department that night; he was X-rayed and given a handful of Percocets for pain and Keflex for infection control. He had wrapped his knees with Ace bandages given to him by a friend, leftovers from an injury that the friend had once sustained. *All I really need*, he said, *is more pain pills.*

I was ready for his request. Pain, now referred to as the fifth vital sign after blood pressure, pulse, respirations, and temperature, is a subjective symptom. Pain exists if the patient says so. Both the Veterans Affairs Administration and the Joint Commission for Accreditation of Health Care Organizations (JCAHO) have proclaimed pain management a necessity in patient care. Pain is to be acknowledged, management implemented, victory declared. Not so simple.

With his history of past drug use (*I did cocaine for about fifteen years; I've been clean for a few months. I just do weed now*), my patient had pain that was complex to manage. Now I recalled John, with his severe osteomyelitis in his ankle and Percocet prescription. With these patients and their interesting pasts involving drug use, I had begun to appreciate that my former naiveté was stunning. Dr. Parks had told me just the day before that he had learned to give a maximum of twelve to fifteen pain pills, narcotics such as Percocet, only if he had hard data, for example, MRI reports. In most cases, he refuses to prescribe narcotics; he also tells his patients up front that he never prescribes Xanax (alprazolam), a short-acting benzodiazepine used to treat anxiety that frequently results in physical dependence. He refers patients to pain-management specialists instead. I took time with my patient to cleanse and dress his multiple gunshot wounds, explaining to him that nonsteroidal anti-inflammatory drugs (NSAIDs), such as ibuprofen, would manage his acute pain better than narcotics. With a reduction in swelling around the nerves trapped in the injured areas, he would experience less pain. I told him that, in fact, NSAIDs were preferable to narcotics in managing pain in tight, enclosed areas, such as in dental surgery and, in his case, with leg trauma. Interestingly, these were not this patient's first gunshot wounds to his legs; an almost same situation occurred four years earlier, at which time a bullet remained lodged behind his left knee. The resultant paraesthesias—numbness and pins-and-needles sensations—in his leg became identified by him as pain. He listened. I gave him sample ibuprofen 400 mg tablets, with instructions to take one to two tablets every six to eight hours for pain as needed, along with food. He said he trusted me. *You're not lying, are you?* I reassured him that I was not lying, and that his past use of recreational drugs could not interfere with his pain management now. He left with instructions to keep his wounds clean, to take the medication as instructed, and to elevate his legs to relief pressure in the wound areas. We threw away his Ace bandages. When he left, I wasn't sure that he would not seek drugs from street dealers; but he had listened, asking questions about what type of foods to take with the ibuprofen to prevent gastritis. Teaching him about alternatives to narcotics for pain relief was rewarding, but it took time. I now wished that Patty, the RN, would always be teamed with me to give care. Together we could treat and teach.

I met my second patient of the day, Shawn, in the waiting room as my first patient hobbled out the door. A fifty-nine-year-old male, extremely quiet, with gentlemanly ways—holding doors, waiting for others to enter rooms before him, shaking hands. I opened his medical record and saw low back pain as his only diagnosis; his medication page listed only acetaminophen for pain, to be taken as needed. *My back pain is gone; the Tylenol worked,* he announced as he sat upright in my chair adjacent to the computer. *What can I do for you today?* He wasn't sure, since he felt better. With a bowed head, he asked if he could have a blood test for hepatitis. He lived in a shelter at night, he explained, and he thought that many of the residents were former drug addicts. *Drug addicts get hepatitis, don't they?*

Given Shawn's past history of alcohol abuse (he had gone through an alcohol rehabilitation program ten years earlier and claimed not to have used alcohol since that time), he was worried that he could get cirrhosis of the liver if he caught hepatitis in the shelter. We reviewed hepatitis; I showed him a website and he read a little about the etiology of the various forms of hepatitis. He had no signs or symptoms of hepatitis, nor did he have any risk factors associated with hepatitis. He could not, however, be dissuaded from his worry. This patient's primary diagnosis at this moment was worry. Worry did not have a CPT code. He was anxious about the possibility of having hepatitis. And while I had assessed him as a reliable narrator of his chief complaint and past medical history, I realized that I may not have received his whole story. Given that he had Medicaid health insurance that covered a hepatitis profile and liver function tests, I ordered these tests, instructing him to return in two weeks to review the results. On the encounter form, I checked anxiety state unspecified—code 300.00—forcing a square peg into a round hole. Often I was unsure if I would see patients for follow-up, but I was very sure that I would see this patient again. Once we developed trust, it is possible that he would give me his whole story. For now, he was a bit of a mystery.

My last patient that same day was Dawn, a thirty-three-year-old female with a past medical history that frightened me—multiple psychiatric diagnoses, including bipolar disorder, major depression, and acute anxiety. (At the end of a busy day, it is tough to have a complex patient, particularly given the amount of documentation required!) She also had hypertension, hypercholesterolemia, gastroesophageal reflux disorder, and obesity. Her electronic medical record—such a great tool to see what is going on quickly!—listed ten current medications. I turned the monitor to her so that she could view it as well. What was her main reason for being here today? (I remembered to *focus*; just remembering this word calmed me down from her expansive list of active medical diagnoses.) *I'm here because you folks gave me this follow-up appointment*, she said with a flat affect.

I took control. Well, your blood pressure is Stage 1 hypertension—do you take your two medications every day for your blood pressure? *No.* Do you take your medication to control your cholesterol? *No.* Do you take any of your medications on this list? *No.* Umm. Are you depressed or sad now? *No more than usual.* Do you feel like you might hurt yourself? *No, I have never wanted to off myself.* Now what? I noted that she had Medicaid health insurance and was eligible for routine blood work. I wasn't sure about how to manage her, so I shut the monitor off and just faced her—chair-to-chair, face-to-face. How do you want us to work together? What do you want to work on yourself? Since she didn't like being sad, she said she was willing to see the psychiatric mental health nurse practitioner when I offered this referral to her. She also wanted to lose weight. She asked me to look at her record again. Had I noticed that she had lost six pounds since her last appointment at the center? Yes, she had lost six pounds. I congratulated her; she told me that she had stopped drinking sodas and had switched to water. Would she be willing to see the nutritionist? She laughed for the first time. *She was a sweet person,* the patient said, *but I can't afford the food she tells me to buy.* She promised to try to remember to write down what she ate each day for the next two weeks—a diet diary, a common means of helping people see their eating patterns. We made a deal—more walking, a mental health referral, and a diet diary. She refused to take any medications; *they get lost in the shelter at night anyway.* She was also willing to have baseline blood work done, so that we could measure improvement over time. When she left, I thought of how unusual this encounter was, so very different from practice in more affluent areas.

As the curtain closed, I rose to meet the verdict. What would a jury of my peers conclude about my management regimen?

North and South: Sustainable Nurse-Managed Primary Care

Frances, said Waldemar "Buzz" Johanson in fall 1998, *you simply cannot do primary care in this place!* Buzz, professor and chairperson of medicine at the University of Medicine and Dentistry of New Jersey (UMDNJ)—New Jersey Medical School, was absolutely exasperated with me and my intent to offer nurse practitioner–managed primary care in community-based organizations in Newark, New Jersey. He stood in the center of the main office of our health center within the Saint Columba Neighborhood Club on Pennsylvania Avenue in Newark and spun around, arms crossed against his chest, critically eyeing our resources—an examination table and stool, metal desk, file cabinet, office supplies, and various clinical supplies. *It can't be done*, he proclaimed, in his heavy Texas accent.

Since New Jersey State Board of Nursing regulations required nurse practitioners to have collaborative practice agreements with licensed physicians in order to practice, I had wanted to establish a relationship with him and, through him, with other physicians within his department. The Board of Nursing regulations required that one or more physicians be available for consultation as needed for the management of complex patients who might require specialty referrals. At the time, the UMDNJ–School of Nursing offered three nurse-managed health centers, two in Newark and one in Camden, where I had practiced primary care upon leaving administration. The Newark centers included one located within the Saint Columba Neighborhood Club (SCNC) on Pennsylvania Avenue, a Hispanic community-based organization, and one in a public housing building adjacent to the university—the New Hope Village center. In Camden, the Community Health Center was located on Broadway, in the heart of the city, within a few blocks of the city's primary acute care hospital, Cooper Hospital University Medical Center.

Nursing's community health center, sponsored collaboratively with the SCNC, was a bustling, thriving wellness center, at one point supported by a major program grant by the Robert Wood Johnson Foundation. Two professional registered nurses, staff within the UMDNJ-School of Nursing, offered several health education programs to local neighborhood residents. From the Baby-Think-It-Over program—a program designed to allow children to experience the demands of infant care with the goal of discouraging teenage pregnancies—to childhood immunizations to exercise classes, residents saw the nurses' services as integral to the offerings provided within the club. While we enjoyed successful outcomes at this center, I remained disappointed. Neither Buzz nor any of his colleagues were willing to serve as collaborating physician for the start-up of a nurse practitioner–managed primary care practice. We offered wellness programs but were walled off from providing primary care in this impoverished neighborhood. Interestingly, to the residents we served our care was stellar; they did not differentiate between primary care and health promotion and disease-prevention efforts. Since the university transportation van service modified their route to include the club, residents were transported to University Hospital or the medical or dental clinics as needed. Residents were satisfied.

Without a demonstration of the nurse practitioner model of primary care, I was, however, disappointed. My profession, I felt, needed to model new ways of providing primary care in neighborhood locales. While I believed that blood work and other diagnostics could be managed via arrangements with outside laboratories and vendors, Buzz wanted them provided on-site—in an ambulatory practice with mauve-colored walls, pastel paintings, new age music or jazz, and a plethora of staff for appointments, billing, and other services. In contrast, I was willing to forgo sophisticated one-stop shopping and provider convenience for sites accessible to residents, even if they needed to go to external agencies for X-rays, blood work, or other diagnostics. Buzz simply would not compromise; thus, the nursing centers in Newark shifted gears to focus on wellness, with our University Hospital assisting us with under-the-table supplies endorsed by the Hispanic chief executive officer.

I learned to become hypervigilant. My experiences with Buzz were simply the beginning of a long series of unsuccessful attempts to collaborate with physicians in Newark or New Brunswick, New Jersey. In addition to the rhetoric about the structure and resources in a primary care practice, there existed an undercurrent of annoyance about nurse practitioners. In the 1990s, my encounters with academic physicians at UMDNJ in Newark proved challenging. In seeking collaboration with psychiatry, I was told that only weak people needed to collaborate; strong people, such as psychiatrists, did not need to collaborate—they were already whole. A pediatric specialist said that he was willing to collaborate with me (that is, nurse practitioners and nurses from the School of Nursing) as long as I returned one-half of every dollar we earned from patient care services to him. In fact, I had offered to pay for his services as a collaborating physician, just simply not that much. Another medical dean, when asked if his medical faculty would serve as preceptors for nurse practitioner students, said no; why would he participate in training the very people who might someday replace physicians? Plus, he could take care of sniffles too, so why shouldn't he get paid for it?

My experiences in Camden, however, were quite different. In southern New Jersey, UMDNJ had two campuses—one in Stratford, a suburb of Camden, and one in Camden. The Stratford campus, housing the Schools of Osteopathic Medicine (SOM) as well as nursing and health-related professions, was anchored by the dean of osteopathy. The dean, a charming, gentle and gracious osteopath and informal provost, had invited other schools to locate on his campus, wishing it to take on the image of an academic health sciences campus. The Camden campus at that time served as a clinical campus for the Robert Wood Johnson Medical School, which had its primary administrative offices in New Brunswick. Osteopaths in Stratford; allopaths in Camden. In the mid-1990s, I developed what would become a lovely working relationship with the dean of SOM and the faculty in the Department of Family Medicine. The SOM dean, whose sister was a nurse practitioner, supported both interdisciplinary education as well as collaborative practice. The chair of Family Medicine signed collaborative practice agreements with several nurse practitioner faculty members who worked in the Camden Community Health Center. Many nursing faculty received reciprocal courtesy faculty appointments to Family Medicine, and the nursing and medical faculty designed and implemented coursework in clinical skills and physical diagnosis. Both faculty groups taught in the same course, each teaching that which they knew best. The relationship between nursing and osteopathic physicians remained solid long after I had left UMDNJ in 2008. Osteopaths and nurse practitioners—neither of whom are at the top of the health sciences hierarchy—shared, I appreciated over time, a common bond, a focus on primary care practice rather than specialty practice. And, since neither group shared allopathic physicians' position of perceived preeminence within the health care system, we were allies. When working in the Camden Community Health Center, I referred uninsured, underinsured, and insured patients to family medicine as needed; these patients were never refused.

Having a sustainable system beyond grants and volunteerism, however, was a challenge both in Camden and Newark. UMDNJ did not include nursing's health centers within their off-campus practice array, citing inability to comply with state regulatory requirements for ambulatory practices at either Pennsylvania Avenue in Newark or Broadway in Camden. Neither center, for example, had handicap access. Additionally, neither center would meet the criteria for designation as a federally qualified health center, given that they belonged to the university—an institution incapable of having a board of trustees with at least 51 percent of its members from the community.

As I worked in Newark to establish a nurse-managed primary care center during the mid-1990s, Nancy Rothman, Elaine Fox, and Tine Hansen-Turton were working to achieve the same goal in Philadelphia. In 1995, Nancy was an associate professor of nursing at Thomas Jefferson University in Center City Philadelphia. Nancy was recruited to Temple through a call for proposals by the Independence Foundation for the establishment of endowed professors of urban community nursing. In 1996, Susan Sherman joined the Independence Foundation as its president and chief executive officer. The foundation is a private, not-for-profit philanthropic organization that supports organizations providing services to people who do not ordinarily have access to them. Such services include health care, legal aid, and social and human services. Susan, a nurse, had served as the chair of the department of nursing at the Community College of Philadelphia for the previous fifteen years. When tapped for the role at the foundation, Susan anticipated the response of the academic nursing community. A community college administrator named as president and CEO of such a prestigious foundation? How could that be? Nursing's elite at the baccalaureate and higher degree-granting institutions were aghast. Susan, however, understood why she was invited to take this position. Simply put, she was good at administration and even better at obtaining and managing money. Susan looked locally within Philadelphia—how could the foundation's money be leveraged to facilitate interaction and synergy among nursing leaders in the city? In 1996, she sent out a Call for Proposals to the eight nursing programs in Philadelphia. She indicated that the foundation sought four leaders to be named Independence Foundation Professors of Urban Community Nursing.

Susan was eager for change. She had an urgency to pull together nursing leaders from diverse sectors to work on a common goal—to improve the health of community residents through quality nursing services. Four Independence Professors were named—Nancy Rothman from Temple University, Lois Evans from the University of Pennsylvania, Katherine Kinsey from LaSalle University, and Elaine Tagliareni from the Community College of Philadelphia. Once named, these four women were charged with the task of presenting a White Paper to the foundation's board on the future of nursing in Philadelphia, on the contributions that nursing could make to improve the health indices of city residents. They recommended a shift in emphasis and resources from acute hospital care to primary health care offered through strong community-provider partnerships. Very importantly, they made concrete, practical suggestions. Data-driven processes and cost-effective nurse-managed models of primary health care needed to be implemented and tested. They concluded that the foundation should support funding cycles that would allow for stabilization and sufficient critical analysis of nurse-managed models of care. Susan encouraged the foundation's funding of nursing centers, pulling these centers together in an organization called the Regional Nursing Centers Consortium. By 2000, the RNCC had gone national, with central offices in Philadelphia and an office in Washington, D.C. The RNCC and its successor organization, the National Nursing Centers Consortium (NNCC), partnered with both Resources for Human Development (RHD) and the Public Health Management Corporation (PHMC) to expand its work and influence.

Knowing that the Independence Foundation's seed funding of the Temple Health Connection—a primary care, nurse-managed health center in North Philadelphia—would eventually end, and that sustainable sources of grant funding were notoriously unpredictable and fragile, Nancy Rothman sold the program to PHMC for one dollar in the early twenty-first century. Since the four centers run by PHMC are designated as federally qualified health centers, their clinical services are reimbursed and administrative services are provided. Once ownership shifted from Temple University to PHMC, the clinical director of the transformed PHMC Health Connection was no longer responsible for credentialing of staff, billing and receiving, and other duties beyond the direct provision of care. The other Philadelphia centers within the PHMC nurse-managed network include the Care Clinic on Callowhill Street, the Mary Howard Health Center on Samson Street, and Rising Sun Health Center on Adams Avenue—all in Philadelphia. Other health centers partnered with RHD for similar services and sustainable income. In 2005, Tine Hansen-Turton assumed an additional responsibility as the PHMC vice president of Health Care Policy and Access; and Nancy, that same year, became funded by PHMC as the director of their Nursing Network. Additionally, Elaine Fox, the PHMC vice president for Specialized Health Services, oversees the health centers in her management portfolio. Through the mutual efforts of Susan, Nancy, Tine, and Elaine, nurse-managed health centers offer primary care services in Philadelphia—and they are reimbursed. An interesting group of dynamic, quietly powerful women, all have links to education, government, and insurers. This group had broken through the morass of nursing's own politics, third-party payers' reticence to cover nurse practitioners as primary care providers, and legislators' ignorance regarding nurse practitioners; physician groups were even willing to serve as collaborating physicians.

Quite impressive. And quite atypical in nursing. The partnership of Susan and Nancy with Tine and Elaine turned the tide. The acknowledgment that nurses need business partners to flourish in practice was wise, and can be attributed to Susan, whom Nancy termed "the matchmaker." As these women formed their own partnership to improve health care through better use of nurses and nurse practitioners, Nancy became increasingly removed from the Temple nursing faculty, of which she was a tenured member. *Yes,* she told me recently, smiling, *I am disconnected from faculty. They seem to think that if you are enjoying yourself, you can't be working hard.* Her work is meaningful and rich in context and diversity. I told her once that I saw her as my stargate, taking liberty with a television show by the same name. Her connections to health care at the local, regional, and state levels are deep and expansive, and she enjoys the respect of all who work with her. At the departmental level, Nancy is peripheral to the core educational work; I think this disconnect is liberating for her. While nursing students may have experiences at the health centers, faculty members are not excited about providing these. Certainly there are compelling reasons for faculty not to engage—too many classes to teach, no reimbursement when serving there, too much committee work, and so on. Some may simply no longer be interested in practice—too tiring, too risky, possible liability. As a profession, nursing disconnects practice from education, with faculty not required to continue practicing as a component of their role. Tenure requirements do not acknowledge practice; in fact, practice draws one away from the incentivized activities for tenure, including grant writing and publication. No wonder Nancy, a tenured full professor at Temple, feels a bit disconnected. She is unsure if she wishes to be designated as a Temple Institute; such a designation may result in institutional taxation. Perhaps remaining outside the walls of the very castle that was unwilling to bring her officially into the health care system as an official unit is wise. In the borderlands, life is contingent.

Patient Protection and Affordable Health Care?

September 23, 2010, marked the six-month anniversary of President Obama's signing of Public Law 111–148: Patient Protection and Affordable Health Care Act. On the eve of this anniversary, the *New York Times* ran an article entitled "For Many, Health Care Relief Begins Today." *The new health care law,* wrote author Kevin Sack, *is expected to bring [profound relief] to hundreds of thousands of Americans who have been stricken first by disease and then by a Darwinian insurance system.* The passage of this act was a wonderful accomplishment, though not what I have been advocating for the past three decades. Many steps in the right direction, yes; a stunning accomplishment, no. The core I demand is universal health care, not peripheral tinkering with health insurance reform. While pleased that the Supreme Court upheld Public Law 111–148 on June 28, 2012, I remain committed to universal health care as a right.

Before Sack wrote about the profound relief anticipated by public law 111–148, President Bill Clinton had passionately told Congress and the American people on September 22, 1993, that "this health care system of ours is badly broken, and it is time to fix it. Our health care is too uncertain and too expensive, too bureaucratic and too wasteful," he claimed, noting that "it has too much fraud and too much greed." Clinton's health care platform aimed at "giving every American health security—health care that can never be taken away, health care that is always there." I watched Bill and Hilary Clinton on television, sitting at the edge of my seat, truly stunned at what I heard, taping the entire speech on my VCR for posterity. I was a believer. I trusted that together they could do it: health care security for every American.

In the spring before Clinton's speech to Congress, I had testified at a local town hall meeting at the University of Medicine and Dentistry of New Jersey (UMDNJ) Robert Wood Johnson Medical School in New Brunswick, New Jersey, about the role nursing could and would play in a reformed health care system. Speaking before Tipper Gore and several members of Clinton's health reform team, I, along with other members of the university's administration, provided input. I still have my testimony notes. I recall vividly how nervous I was that day, even what I wore—a suit with a pin of an American flag on the collar. Nurses, I had testified, needed to move from being the invisible background of the system to the front door—to serve as primary care providers, to promote healthy lifestyles. Nurses were an army of highly skilled providers, with various skill sets capable of ensuring an efficient and financially sound system of care, providers who would call in specialists as warranted.

In the seventeen intervening years between the Clinton and the Obama presidencies, I have remained in health care as an administrator, teacher, and nurse practitioner. Graduating in May 1998 as an adult nurse practitioner from the UMDNJ School of Nursing—the very program I had created in 1990—I continued to provide primary care in the fast-track emergency department of University Hospital in Newark on a part-time basis, while my primary position was that of a faculty administrator. Once I moved to Temple University in 2008, I was fortunately able to continue to practice as a nurse practitioner at the Mary Howard Health Center in Philadelphia.

Health care looks different from the street level. The daily business of doing health care, the volume of patients to treat, the time constraints, the need for accurate documentation, the diversity of referral protocols and medication approvals required for third-party payers, and the sheer need to keep up with information on diseases and management alternatives are enormous responsibilities. Often, we lack time to do the single most important intervention—teaching patients to manage their illness and to improve their lifestyles. Delivering care can be tiring, particularly in patient populations with multiple comorbidities and poverty.

During these years, I have become more pragmatic, more willing to accept the frailties of our health care system and the real providers who compose it. While still optimistic about change in our system, I have now allowed myself to see the dark side. As President Clinton said, our system is fraught with greed. Simple contrasts between ambulatory-practice offices of nurse-managed health centers that serve poor patients and those managed by physician practices that serve more affluent populations—provide evidence of income. In recent years, concierge or boutique medicine—highly personalized care for patients who pay an annual fee and receive individualized care, including access to their physician's home phone number—has taken root in wealthy communities. I have learned to appreciate the enormous pushback force of our capitalistic system—the intense desire for wealth that deeply, and often quite invisibly, imbalances our society's intent to provide care for all. I doubt that greed can be eradicated.

Compounding greed is another equal and opposing force—ennui, a sense of boredom and listlessness about changing the system. Shifting the paradigm from the current payer system to one of universal access upsets not only capitalism, but also complacency. While Nancy, Tine, Elaine, and Susan advocate for a nursing model of care, the majority of nurses are educated at the associate-degree level with only a minority engaged in their state's professional organization. Most are employed by hospitals, where nursing services are billed as a part of a bundled charge. In contrast, nurse practitioners, prepared at the graduate-degree level, are termed primary care provider (PCP), as are their medical, osteopathy, midwifery, and physician assistants colleagues. Despite this situation, however, as Ariel Levy points out in her article "Life and Separate" in the *New Yorker* (November 16, 2009), "preoccupation with representation suggests that feminism has lost its larger ambitions."

Is it enough to have the label, or does having the label *PCP* mandate even more courage, more change? As Tine Hansen-Turton said in August 2010, nurse practitioners need to *focus, focus, focus*, on reimbursement issues, policy, and politics. She fears the nurse practitioner movement has plateaued; I fear it may take a different road from primary care.

Satisfied with the accomplishment of the PCP designation, many nurse practitioners now specialize, following their medical colleagues in the path away from primary care into the more lucrative areas, serving as sophisticated assistants to medical specialists. Doctor of Nursing Practice (DNP) programs—clinical doctorates originally designed to prepare primary care providers to practice evidence-based care—now offer tracks in education, in informatics, in administration. In a general faculty meeting in October 2010 at Temple, I noted that our draft DNP program outcomes looked more like objectives for degree programs in public policy, public health, or public administration than for a program in direct primary care. Are we moving down a road of liberal arts—studying questions of health care rather than direct provision of primary care—to mainstream nursing as an academic discipline? We eventually reframed our objectives to reflect a primary care focus; however, reframing takes energy, political courage, and time. It is easier to regress toward mediocrity than to remain an outlier pushing for change. Employment as a physician's nurse practitioner in specialty care may, in fact, have more attractive and tangible benefits than providing care in a nursing center—higher salary, less risk (complex cases are quickly triaged to medicine), stable hours.

Sometimes while I am on a SEPTA subway going to the Mary Howard Center, I think of a core problem: the conflict between focusing on a patient's chief complaint versus focusing on the patient's more complex presentation that impacts his or her health status. There is no reimbursement for managing illiteracy and lack of education with a prescription to matriculate in a community college. But yet, given the multidimensionality of health, poverty and ignorance are deeply enmeshed as factors related to poor health indices. Our care system simply cannot deal with the complexities of health. Our reimbursement system, a modern era symbol of capitalism, reinforces and rewards an illness paradigm.

Irrespective of these dark thoughts, however, nurse practitioner change agents do exist. And 111–148 provides windows for improved health delivery services. Section 5208 nurse-managed health clinics provides for funding to centers managed by advanced practice nurses who serve vulnerable or underserved populations. I find it telling that such grants will be targeted to our vulnerable citizens; in the twenty-first century, our vulnerable citizens—often the sickest in our system—are served by nurse practitioners. I am part of a two-tiered system.

It is reminiscent of an experience in my UMDNJ past. When the nurse practitioners in the School of Nursing developed a Student Health Center for all students on the Newark campus in the mid-1990s, an associate dean of the medical school sent his students the following comment: *Medical students to receive second-class care by second-class providers in a second-class center.* Shortly thereafter, the Student Health Center was put under the umbrella of the medical school, to the relief of medical students and faculty. The Community Health Center, offered as a collaborative venture with the community-based Hispanic organization, the Saint Columba's Neighborhood Club, remained under the sole auspices of the School of Nursing. And, since it only received interest income from a Hearst Foundation endowment, it offered shoestring services to underinsured or uninsured local residents, referred if needed to the medical school's clinics. On a micro- or macrolevel, an interesting caste system survives. On a realistic note, such funding did enable nurse practitioners to service those without primary care access; thus, applying for such funding will be a priority for those involved with vulnerable populations.

With effort, the two-tiered system can be reconceptualized. In fall 2010, faculty in Temple's Department of Nursing began offering school-nurse services in a new public charter school in north Philadelphia—the Pan American Academy. This charter school opened in fall 2008, accepting students from kindergarten through fourth grade. The Academy's focus is on inquiry-based learning, with the mission to prepare the next generation of strong, internationally minded leaders in our community. With a grant from the National Nursing Centers Consortium to implement this program, the department provided nurse practitioner staff to meet the standard school-nurse functions and to evolve the services into a full primary care center. Since the Academy is aligned with Congreso de Latinos Unidos, a community-based human services organization located less than one mile away, it is part of a larger organization caring for the complex needs of this North Philadelphia population. The Public Health Management Corporation (PHMC), working with Congreso, anticipates opening a federally qualified primary care health center at its site on Somerset Street. Thus, once the Academy school nurse services transition to primary care services for children and their families, then cooperation between Congreso and the wellness Center at Pan American Academy will allow for richer, more robust health services delivery at this very local level. The nursing faculty will then expand their services as PCPs under PHMC's structure, delivering care and teaching at the point of contact of children and their families. Once funded, this model will allow for on-site immunizations of children and immediate primary care delivery in schools, resulting in fewer classroom absences, and, perhaps, improved health and educational outcomes.

Hierarchy notwithstanding, the Supreme Court's ruling to uphold Public Law 111–148 allows goal-oriented politically adept nurse practitioners to advance their roles in society. The caste system remains all too real, and nurse practitioners remain a part of that reality, edging their presence toward the center.

Chapter 3

Nurse, Are You a Doctor?

Engaging in the quiet privilege that is primary care evolved battles over several decades. Victories, losses, and compromises with physicians, physician assistants, nurses, and administrators constituted the backdrop of my career. Nurse practitioners gained authority to practice through legislation, and legislation is not an activity for the meek. Lobbying to garner legislators' support, nurse practitioners advanced their scope of practice. Physicians' more powerful counterlobbying force mandated, and continues to mandate, sustained hypervigilance by nurses as we counter the forces of power, money, and greed that threaten our entrance into primary care. Unable to defeat the nurse practitioner movement and its ability to provide services at lower health care costs, medicine's efforts have shifted to control nurse practitioner practice through regulations that constrain, limit, and otherwise obscure full independent primary care practice by nurse practitioners. Compromises between nursing and medicine to ensure incremental gains for nurse practitioner practice have resulted in cross-referenced regulations within state boards of nursing and boards of medical examiners that place limits on that very practice. Given nursing's century-old history of control by hospitals and physician expectations of obedient subservience, efforts to limit nurse practitioner practice were certainly not unexpected. What I never anticipated was a backlash from nursing itself. Nurses testified against nurse practitioner practice at public hearings. Nurses bristled against working with nurse practitioners in practice settings. I watched as our profession

oppressed its own members. Then, as in all good stories, support came from unexpected sources.

*

Scrub the area, Marta barked at me. The area was a 2.5-centimeter laceration over the left eyebrow of a twenty-three-year-old male patient. He had been struck in several locations with a baseball bat in a gang fight at the intersection of Springfield Avenue and Irvine Turner Boulevard in Newark. Brought in by the police, he remained feisty even after sedation. On the outside corner of his right eye, he had a tattoo of a teardrop, a symbol, he told me, that he had scored one for his gang in the recent past—his present street battle a retaliation fight for his past victory.

It was about 9 P.M. on a Saturday evening in the emergency department of University Hospital in Newark. The fast-track service closed at 10 P.M., with all patients admitted between that time and 7 A.M. triaged to the main room—the big room—usually reserved for more serious trauma or severe medical problems. With the heavy aroma of the staff's garlic and onion pizza lingering in the air of the fast-track suite, I was nauseous, exhausted, with the early signs of a migraine headache emerging. My young patient was daunting. Still a postmaster's student in the University of Medicine and Dentistry of New Jersey's nurse practitioner program, I would soon be going home after a twelve-hour shift. We were in a patient room littered with debris from servicing previous patients, sticky countertops and scattered empty four-by-four-inch-sponge dressing boxes—these sponges being one of the most commonly used items in patient care. It had been a busy early spring day in the fast track. But Marta was present. A physician's assistant, Marta was experienced, and not shy about her skills. I had learned early on in my rotation in the fast track—I was there every Saturday for twelve hours for two years—that Marta was excellent at surgical procedures, management of sexually transmitted infections, and differential diagnoses. Marta also liked to teach. *See one, do one, teach one*: the axiom often quoted in medical education.

This evening Marta asked the nurse to gather supplies for me, including sterile saline, a basin, more sponges, suture materials, and a Betadine-impregnated surgical scrub brush. Announcing that *my patients' wounds never get infected*, Marta supervised my preparation of the laceration prior to suturing it. First, block the area with a Lidocaine injection, an anesthetic. Then, manually remove any debris in the laceration, including skin tissue and any baseball bat fragments or dirt. Finally, vigorously scrub the area with the betadine scrub brush. An antiseptic, betadine is a common solution used for this purpose. A dark amber color that stains skin, the betadine is then rinsed away with a sterile saline solution. We were quite short-staffed that evening, so the patient served as my assistant, holding an emesis basin to collect the saline as it spilled from the wound. I then sutured the laceration, slowly, carefully, under the intense focused light of the large wall-mounted surgical gooseneck lamp that seemingly burned my retinas. With Marta as supervisor and the patient as assistant, the task was completed—he went to jail with instructions to his police escort to return him the next day for follow-up. I went home.

Ourselves among Others

Physicians' assistants and nurse practitioners, in the 1990s referred to as physician extenders, have become, in the early twenty-first century, widely accepted and integrated into the health care system, each with a scope of practice codified in legislation and delineated in regulations. Each state, however, has its own legislation and regulations for their practice. Powerful lobbying of legislators by state medical societies, sometimes accompanied by support for hospital associations, stalled the emergence of these providers in New Jersey and Pennsylvania for years. Critical also in impeding the use of these providers was the animosity between them and the warfare they waged on each other, adding fuel to delays created by medicine's lobbyists. Although there is enough illness in the United States to warrant an all-hands-on-deck orientation, medicine's fear of loss of income, control, and power, coupled with nursing's fear of competition by physician's assistants, stalled legislation for years. With providers focusing only on themselves and their professional agendas, patients' needs in this game were sidelined. Patients' voices were heard last—or not at all—in such practitioner wars.

As I worked alongside Marta in the fast track, I appreciated the role of the physician assistant (PA) from a very personal perspective. The PA, with a toolkit of surgical and diagnostic skills, practices within the medical model, a disease management orientation. Very highly skilled, Marta truly extends medical care on behalf of her supervising physician. In contrast, the nurse practitioner (NP) practices within a health model, diagnosing and managing disease, but with an orientation toward wellness and healthy lifestyles. While both manage illness, the PA does so as a direct assistant to the physician, and the NP does so as a primary care provider of the patient.

In my role as founding dean of nursing at the University of Medicine and Dentistry of New Jersey, I engaged in marvelous political experiences over many years; ultimately, battles over licensure of physician's assistants and nurse practitioners were the most provocative, marred with some of humans' most basic traits—greed and the desire for power. Without any formal training in negotiation and compromise, I became involved in an engaging, meaningful political situation that drove dramatic change in patient care. It was a thrilling decade. The stage for this legislation had been set in 1990 when James E. McGreevey, chair of the state's Health Care Policy Study Commission, recommended a shift of focus from illness care to health promotion and disease prevention, recognizing that health was less costly than illness. Capitalizing on the chaos and debate engendered by this group, Governor James Florio subsequently appointed the Commission on Health Care Costs in 1990. The commissioners went rogue, urging the use of less-costly providers: nurse practitioners and physician assistants. They demanded that these providers be licensed in New Jersey. The bell had rung, the match begun; physicians in one corner, nurses in the other, with patients in the stands as onlookers.

As with most major efforts, many people were involved, with only a few providing true leadership. Two such leaders emerged in this PA-NP legislative war. One, Stanley S. Bergen Jr., a physician and president of the University of Medicine and Dentistry of New Jersey (UMDNJ); and the other, Andrea Aughenbaugh, chief executive officer of the New Jersey State Nurses Association (NJSNA). They were my mentors for years. Despite past scrimmages, some culminating in court battles, NJSNA and UMDNJ joined forces to move the PA-NP causes forward in 1990. *If we don't move these two bills together, they don't go at all*, proclaimed Stanley. Urging nurse practitioners and physician's assistants to join forces against a more powerful and rich enemy—medicine— Stanley eliminated much of the squabble in the ring. United, the two groups lobbied legislatures. A first effort was to understand the scope of practice of each group—the functions identified as being within their authority to implement, based on educational preparation. Stanley called early morning meetings of the nursing and physician's assistant faculty groups. Within the university's School of Health Related Professions, programs for the preparation of nurse practitioners and physician assistants had been established, in 1990 and 1974, respectively. While it was a forced courtship, the group developed relationships, with a common foe identified. Fact sheets were written, focusing on the education, practice functions, credentialing, and practice privileges specific to nurse practitioners, physician's assistants, allopathic physicians, and osteopathic physicians across the country. The differences among the groups in terms of practice functions were not dramatically different.

Stanley's early morning meetings in his conference room, adjacent to his office in the administrative complex, glued nurse practitioners and physician's assistants together in a cause. The administrative complex was a series of Quonset huts; prefabricated corrugated steel buildings interconnected in a series of eighteen buildings—commonly called the blue buildings. In one of our morning fact-finding sessions—with rain loudly reverberating off the roof, almost too noisy for us to concentrate—our analysis revealed a 70 percent redundancy in practice functions across all groups. The core functions of primary care—services provided by a first-contact provider who diagnoses and either gives the care needed or refers patients to specialists for further management—were shared among physicians, nurse practitioners, and physician's assistants. We had more similarities in practice than we had realized—all were educated to serve as primary care providers. A major difference among the four groups is the board within the New Jersey Division of Consumer Affairs that regulates each group's practice. Nurse practitioners are licensed under the Board of Nursing; physician's assistants, allopathic physicians, and osteopathic physicians are licensed under the Board of Medical Examiners. A physician's assistant extends the supervising physician's capacity to manage a patient caseload, much like a nursing assistant, who provides nursing care to patients under the supervision of a registered nurse.

Our concrete, objective, and practical fact sheet provided a useful tool in achieving our goal. In a total quality management seminar in the early 1990s, I had heard the expression "In God We Trust, All Others Bring Data"; our fact sheet was golden, all data, all objective, with practice functions and educational requirements clearly outlined. Beyond emotion, beyond subjectivity. Legislators ask practical questions, usually questions about money or how an action might negatively impact their chances for reelection. For some, the matter of supporting nurse practitioners was a complex one, given that many of their constituents were nurses, but some of their financial supporters were physicians. Votes versus money. One bitterly cold day in December, I gingerly walked down the wide marbled hallways of the state capitol, deeply impressed by the gilded inner rotunda underneath the golden crown dome. Originally built in 1792, when New Jersey became the third state in the union, the capitol building underwent a major expansion with renovations in 1845, housing offices for the governor, assemblymen, and senators. It is meticulously managed, with a fresh, clean aroma filling the air, quite inconsistent with the building's age. The power in the air was as palpable as the aroma was fresh. Here was where change could germinate. I met with two legislators and their aides that day, lobbying for their support of licensure for nurse practitioners and physician's assistants and answering the most common question: What is the difference between a nurse practitioner and a physician's assistant?

Wynona Lipman, representing the Twenty-ninth Legislative District in the New Jersey senate, had initiated legislation in 1986 to provide nursing specialists with prescriptive powers, a bill that was quite unsuccessful that year (Senate Bill No. 2721). Senator Lipman, however, was tenacious and a friend to Stanley and UMDNJ. She reintroduced her bill (Senate Bill No. 1018) in 1988 and her colleague John Kelly introduced a companion bill in the assembly (Assembly Bill No. 1600) concurrently. Assemblywoman Ann Mullen, from the state's Fourth Legislative District covering municipalities in Camden County, introduced legislation authorizing licensure of physician's assistants in the state—the PA bill.

During this period in the late twentieth century, UMDNJ offered academic programs that prepared graduates to serve in roles for which the state did not yet allow them to practice. I recall thinking at the time that UMDNJ was a missionary institution, graduating nurse practitioners and physician's assistants to work in other states where licensure laws allowed them to practice. It was such a bizarre situation, created by medicine's stranglehold on the entire health care system. To be on the inside of this debacle was interesting—it was absolutely expected that medicine would take the helmet-down, lancets-up posture of battle. Thus, all of our behaviors normalized, with nursing and physician's assistant faculty members, and indeed the university's own president—a physician—strategizing on tactics that would tip the balance of power toward us, thus allowing legislation to pass to allow non-physician providers to practice in the state. No one expected rational behavior from physicians; no one even attempted to neutralize this enemy. Instead, it was a given—medicine would galvanize their power, influence, and money to prevent others from providing primary care in New Jersey. We focused our energy on legislators. They needed to be convinced; they needed to be educated; they also needed to be infused with courage. For knowledge, we gave them data; for courage, we gave them comparisons, focusing on New Jersey's unique status as an outlier state on these issues. How far from the norm did New Jersey wish to be regarding use of nurse practitioners and physician's assistants?

In my earlier practice life as a young critical care nurse working the night shift at the East Orange Veterans Administration Hospital, this squabbling over ownership of primary care words such as diagnosis, treatment, and patient did not touch me. Caring for veterans at night, traveling in the daytime to New York University and attending graduate classes, I was quite oblivious to early skirmishes involving language and payment. I loved NYU. I was thrilled to take the PATH train from Harrison to Ninth Street in New York, walking the few blocks to Washington Square Park, getting coffee at Grestide's supermarket,

and nestling into "my" seat in an old, un-air-conditioned classroom in Shim-
kin Hall on Fourth Street. I had graduated from Rutgers University, College of
Nursing, on the Newark campus in 1972, with a high grade point average and
an intense desire to cure the ills of my city—Newark. While I learned skills at
Rutgers, I became educated at NYU. NYU welcomed all thoughts—indeed, it
seemed that there really was no thought you couldn't think, all ideas worthy of
exploration. I most enjoyed graduate courses in cognitive development, psychometrics, research methods, and test and scale construction—courses involving
theory evolution, the differences between concepts and constructs, the nuances
of language, and paradigms. It was at NYU that I began to appreciate the subtle-
ties of language, the impact of paradigms on daily behavior, and the driving
force of shared values walling out anomalies. It was there that I recognized that
change, on any scale, is difficult. Walking through the park on my way back to
the PATH train and my night-owl life, with the faint hint of marijuana wafting
in the air, I remember realizing that I was beginning to broadly understand how
things might work. My father, an uneducated carpenter who had immigrated to
the United States shortly after World War II, had always said that whatever was
worth doing was worth doing well. He was right. Armed with my toolkit from
Rutgers, my registered nurse license, and my rich understanding acquired from
an array of diverse mentors at NYU, I was prepared to see issues in my field,
and to recognize the pan-dimensionality of debates that were evolving over
constructs such diagnosis, primary care, and prescriptive authority. Rutgers
had taught me answers; NYU stimulated me to question. Once one is taught to
question, it is impossible to return to obedient compliance. By 1975, my world
seemed different. As a young child, my oldest daughter Katie said that she
couldn't sleep again once her eyes had opened. So too with me.

In the twenty or so years intervening between the establishment of physician assistant and nurse practitioner programs and the introduction of legislation licensing these providers, nurses and physicians fought passionately
about primary care—who could provide it, who was educated adequately to
give it, who could be reimbursed for providing it. Primary care brings, as the
World Health Organization states, cure and care together. Primary care means
the diagnosis and management of disease, as well as the promotion of health
and the restoration of well-being. Primary care providers are the front door
to health care; they provide management of common acute illnesses such as
sore throats and urinary tract infections and chronic illnesses such as emphy-
sema, hypertension, and diabetes. Trusting relationships develop between primary care providers and their patients. I trust my patient John who I described
in chapter 2; I acknowledge his complaints of pain and we manage his pain

together. When his pain is too complex for the two of us to manage, I refer him to a pain management specialist. Management of primary care is the financial bread-and-butter of medicine. Providers are reimbursed according to the ICD code linked to any particular disease. Income, linked to ICD code billing, depends on a thriving primary care practice, if one is not a medical specialist. As a dean of one of the UMDNJ medical schools said to me early on in the debate over primary care ownership, *If we [physicians and nurse practitioners] can both bill for sniffles, then why would I not stop you from practicing?* And, more to the point, another medical faculty member promised that he would do whatever it takes to stop nurse practitioners from practicing in New Jersey. The line drawn in the sand was not about quality care, it was solely about income.

So between 1974 and 1990, much angst, like water tumbling over Niagara Falls, was expended. When reports of the high costs of health care, particularly those associated with New Jersey's charity care program, became threatening, there was renewed interest in legislating nurse practitioner and physician's assistants practice. Clearly, time had passed, Bill Clinton was campaigning for president on a health care reform platform, and the shortage of primary care physician providers was only increasing. The crisis resurfaced, again and again. Nursing had united with medicine to prevent legalization of physician's assistants in New Jersey; nursing also battled within its own organizations about the need for separate legislation authorizing nurse practitioners with prescriptive authority. Some on the Board of Nursing advanced the idea that the 1974 amended Nursing Practice Act was all that was needed, that this provided the authority for nurses to engage in expanded practice, including writing prescriptions. They believed it foolish to kowtow to the demands of others. On the other side, UMDNJ, the New Jersey State Nurses Association, and others acknowledged that the matter was conceptually complex, mandating careful placement of words such as diagnosis, management, and prescriptive authority in further amendments to the nursing act. Ownership of words, with the richness of their meanings, was the essential next step.

Senator Lipman met with members of both the New Jersey State Nurses Association and UMDNJ in January 1989, extending an olive branch, urging all present—including me—to make it work for patients. Wynona Lipman was an impressive woman. Her Georgian drawl never faded, despite her years in New Jersey. Her quiet demeanor and unassuming comportment understated her knowledge and skills. Articulate to a fault but unaggressive in her speech, Wynona, who earned her PhD from Columbia University, played her political cards extremely well. I recall that she first just let everyone speak, then she asked us to make it work for patients. For many years she was the sole black person and only woman in the New Jersey Senate, a body she called the men's club. The university's three medical schools opposed her bill; the University Hospital and College of Health Related Professions supported the bill, as did the nursing association. Stanley Bergen, the university president, announced that the university would support the bill, as long as the PA and NP bills were considered simultaneously. A leader. In effect, he silenced his internal opposition, setting the stage to win both the PA and the NP bills together. And, while we all knew that the medical schools were still privately opposed, we also knew that they would not go public and oppose the bills.

In an interesting afternoon, I found myself alone with Senator Lipman in Stanley Bergen's Quonset hut conference room. She wanted me to help her understand why physicians were so strongly opposed to her bill. We looked again at the Fact Sheet; I reviewed nurse practitioner education as well as physician's assistant education. We compared education across the disciplines of medicine, osteopathy, nurse practitioner, and physician's assistant in terms of hours of clinical pharmacology, management of disease, physical examination and history taking techniques, differential diagnosis, physiology and pathophysiology, amount of clinical experiences with patients, and other features for comparison. To be a nurse practitioner, you need first to be a licensed registered nurse. In addition, you must have graduate education in advanced nursing practice, including supervised clinical practice, pharmacology, and patient follow-up. Physician's assistants are trained in the medical model to extend medical management, particularly disease management. Their education is not built on an earlier license; this is their sole educational program. She took me as an expert. I felt confident, from my years of health care experiences, that I knew what to include in legislation for nurse practitioners. She gave me a copy of her bill and asked that I revise it. A truly thrilling experience! With her request, Wynona opened the door for me to work directly with Andrea Aughenbaugh, the chief executive officer of the New Jersey State Nurses Association. After we agreed to several iterations over many phone calls and meetings, the language of the bill became acceptable to both UMDNJ and NJSNA.

The hours of compromising and negotiating on the Lipman bill paid off. On January 15, 1992, both the nurse practitioner bill and the PA bill were signed into law (Chapter 377, *Laws of New Jersey*, 1991) by Governor James J. Florio. It was a beginning. But as Stanley Bergen wrote on the card inside a bouquet of red roses given to me by the UMDNJ deans to celebrate this victory, *remember that the snakes are still in the grass!*

He was, of course, right. Passage of the law won us the right to battle more. To pass the bill, compromises similar to the ones crafted in other states' bills had to be made. Andrea was my rock through all of this. As the chief executive officer of the state's nursing association, Andrea had to deal with a host of nursing constituencies, all with different, and, at times, competing, agendas. With silver hair, a slow and easy Texas-sounding drawl, the petite-sized Andrea was patient and always willing to discuss and compromise. Andrea was keenly aware that she represented all nurses in the state and she was a serious, and fair, executive. She appreciated that the two bills—the nurse practitioner and the physician's assistant bills—needed to be more similar than dissimilar in order to be passed by the legislature. I learned patience from Andrea. *Change is incremental*, she said. Like it or not, nursing gains in scope of practice were won primarily in legislation, not through education. And, since our gains were often perceived by medicine and hospital administrators as their losses, we needed to prove that each incremental gain did not result in harm to the public. For each gain, time had to pass, data had to be amassed, and patient outcomes needed to be proved positive before the next gain was won. Andrea was politically savvy, as was Stanley Bergen. Both understood that fast, sweeping changes to the Nursing Practice Act, first passed in 1903 in New Jersey (Chapter 109), were impossible. Winning allies to incremental changes, neutralizing some potential enemies, and squaring off openly with foes (with data in hand!) has historically been the process used to amend nurses' scope of practice. This was particularly true in 1991 in the effort to give nurse practitioners prescriptive authority.

Scope of Practice

Public law 1991, chapters 377 and 378, defines the requirements for nurse practitioners and physician's assistants, respectively. Chapter 377 enables nurse practitioners to manage preventive care services and diagnose and manage deviations from wellness and long-term illnesses, consistent with the needs of the patient. This legislation dramatically expanded nurses' legal scope of practice. It allowed nurse practitioners to diagnose disease and to treat it with drugs and other therapies. Diagnose—a word historically ascribed to medicine. In the 1980s, nursing adopted this word and began a movement to assign nursing diagnoses to patients' conditions, with corollary nursing interventions prescribed for management—a rather lame attempt to demonstrate that the word "diagnosis" was not owned by medicine. While less in vogue currently, nursing diagnosis language still exists, found frequently in undergraduate course syllabi and in hospital nursing-care plans. I had always found nursing diagnosis language to be offensive, a Mickey Mouse version of the diagnostic codes used by medicine for reimbursement for services by health insurance companies.

In practical terms, Chapter 377 gave nurse practitioners a much widened scope of practice—a phrase used to denote the specific functions that practitioners could perform. Encroaching on medicine's traditional tasks, these functions included initiating laboratory and other diagnostic tests, prescribing or ordering medications and devices, and prescribing or ordering treatments, including referrals to other health care providers. To move the bill, a major compromise had been needed to get physicians on board and thus allow legislators supported by physicians to relax their opposition. This compromise cloaked the reality that physicians were ultimately still in control. The control mechanism, in this case, was the collaborative practice agreement, a document detailing joint protocols for practice mutually accepted by the nurse practitioner and collaborating physician. Politically, the requirement to establish joint protocols was brilliant. Since cardiac monitoring in intensive care units was instituted in the 1960s, nurses trained in coronary care used standing orders to administer specific drugs and treatments to prevent complications and/or sudden death from arrhythmias in heart attack patients. Standing orders are written instructions from a physician enabling nurses to administer drugs and/or treatments to patients evidencing specific objective findings without a prescription. Such orders are commonplace in acute care hospitals. If a patient develops a sudden ventricular tachycardia, noted in the cardiac monitor, then the nurse may deliver a certain predetermined dose of Lidocaine intravenously. If a kidney failure patient develops nausea and vomiting while on peritoneal dialysis, then Compazine pills or suppositories may be given, if the patient's blood pressure is normal. The mandate to require collaborative practice agreements evolved naturally from the standing orders of the past. And, since these agreements required negotiation between the nurse practitioner and the physician, they approached the team concept. Orders, on the other hand, imply compliance and obedience.

Shortly after passage of this legislation, I hosted a meeting of the baccalaureate and higher degree nursing program deans and directors to discuss the standards for joint protocols to be adopted by the director of the Division of Consumer Affairs. The university frequently held meetings in a spacious office building in New Brunswick, immediately off the New Jersey Turnpike and adjacent to Route 18 in the central section of the state. I was nervous. Knowing that the snakes were still in the grass, and that the university's three medical schools harbored physicians unhappy about nurse practitioner gains, I wanted nursing school administrators to rally to the cause in a united way. My goal was to develop draft standards for joint protocols that the group would forward to the director for his use in discussions with the nursing and medical boards. I have always believed in the power of the pen. If you are willing to write, then it is highly probable that your language will influence the final outcome.

What occurred that day still stuns me, all these years later. We were at a long conference table, with all participants having been provided a packet of information on the legislation. Quiet, absolute, uneasy quiet. Palpable discomfort prevailing. A click of a pen, a cough—the only sounds present at the beginning of the meeting. Representing deans and directors of baccalaureate and graduate programs in the state, this group was primarily suspicious of my motives and accusatory in tone. While I knew that the new president of the Board of Medical Examiners was a university physician uncomfortable with the legislative progress of nurse practitioners in the state, these nursing faculty administrators saw me as their primary problem. Several indicated that nurses had enjoyed wider scopes of practice before the legislation had passed, that all nurses could previously engage in primary care practice. Now, some claimed, due to the compromises made in legislation, only nurse practitioners could write prescriptions, where previously the nursing practice act allowed all nurses to enjoy this privilege. I was seen as an enemy—the single nurse in the state viewed as a quisling working on behalf of medicine, given my appointment to the University of Medicine and Dentistry of New Jersey. One had even called me, in a national nursing conference, the brain-dead pawn of the university's president, Stanley Bergen.

The ignorance of the specifics of Chapter 377 revealed during that meeting was an epiphany—a true wake-up call to me regarding nursing's intraprofessional oppression and internal wars. I recall going home that day thinking of a dean's meeting earlier that year when an opportunity to manage a new statewide clinical initiative in correctional health was discussed. All of the deans wanted a piece of this initiative to control; I was no different. One medical school dean assured me, however, that nursing could not participate simply because *we could never get our act together on anything important.* Nursing was thus dismissed as a potential player in the effort. I thought, with regret, that my medical colleagues were correct; nurses would not pose a threat to physicians' statewide control of correctional health.

I found myself aligning with Andrea Aughenbaugh, both for mentorship and for validation of my beliefs. Under Andrea's leadership, the standards for joint protocols were eventually adopted. A simple set of rules, joint protocols, were to be written, published, reviewed on a regular basis, housed in practice locations, and included in collaborative practice agreements. The deed was done, completed not by academic leaders, but by an expert in compromise. Historically, nursing evolved outside the higher education arena, with gains in practice accrued through legislation rather than through degree attainment, a testament to workforce mentality imposed on nursing by medicine and hospitals. Indeed, to be licensed as a registered nurse in New Jersey, as in most states, one has simply to be educated in a hospital diploma school, a community college, or a four-year college or university. A nurse is a nurse, without differentiation by education.

Certification as a nurse practitioner is dependent on certification by a voluntary professional organization. Unlike the physician's assistant, the nurse practitioner must first hold current licensure as a registered professional nurse. Nurse practitioners can be certified to practice based on criteria published by one of several voluntary professional organizations. The American Nurses Credentialing Corporation, a subsidiary of the American Nurses Association, provides credentialing programs in several specialty practice areas, including adult and family nurse practitioners. A second organization, the American Academy of Nurse Practitioners credentials adult, gerontological, and family nurse practitioners. Each of these organizations publishes very specific criteria that must be met in order to sit for the board certification requested. Once certified, the nurse practitioner completes the process to be certified by the board of nursing in the state in which she or he wishes to work. Board certification must be renewed every five years, with renewal based on successfully meeting renewal criteria, including hours of practice and number of continuing education credits attained, including a certain number in pharmacologic management. I have found these processes and requirements quite minimalist. Given my love of continuing education, meeting the number of credits required is quite easy to meet, and exceed. In my last renewal cycle, I had over two hundred continuing education credits, far exceeding the number required. Perhaps these confessions are best left unrecorded.

The New Jersey State Board of Nursing (BON) issues certification to practice as an advanced practice nurse to registered professional nurses who are at least eighteen years of age with good moral character, who have completed an educational program including pharmacology that has been approved by the board, and who have passed a written examination approved by the board. The requirement of a good moral character is operationalized by criminal background checks and drug screening conducted by schools both prior to, and throughout, educational programs. The BON accepts applications for certification from registered nurses who have passed an examination in their clinical specialty that was developed by a national certifying agency accredited by either the American Board of Nursing Specialties and/or the National Commission for Certifying Agencies. While any new educational program leading to licensure as a registered professional nurse—a hospital diploma program, a community college associate degree program, or a baccalaureate degree program—must undergo review and approval by the BON prior to entering a first class, any new graduate program leading to certification as a nurse practitioner must be reviewed and approved only by the state's Commission on Higher Education. Programs leading to RN licensure undergo additional review by the BON, a state agency mandated to assure the public's safety. In designing a nurse practitioner graduate education program, templates for structure, content, and evaluation are provided by the professional certification organizations—a loop that begins with the organization's recipe for an educational program and ends with certification awarded by that organization.

I joined the University of Medicine and Dentistry of New Jersey as the chair of the Department of Nursing Education and Services in 1986, during a period of national debate about how many hours of continuous hospital service are deemed safe for medical residents in acute care hospitals. Residents, or graduate medical students working under direct supervision by an attending physician, often work excessively long hours, sometimes ending their shifts in an operating room or in emergency room trauma bay—at a time when they may be dramatically sleep deprived. When viewed as an educational experience, the care delivered by medical residents requires oversight, validation, and review by attending-physician educators. As cheap labor, residents put in long hours; their hours have stirred debate in the medical education community for years. In 1999, the National Labor Relations Board rendered a decision holding resident physicians to be employees of teaching hospitals, thereby able to unionize and bargain collectively for rights, privileges, and benefits. It was much later—in 2007—that the Accreditation Council for Graduate Medical Education approved duty hours' language in the learning and working environment. Residency hours are a hot topic, somewhat analogous to nursing's early days of 24/7 subservience in hospital training schools, environments in which they lived, worked, and toiled with minimum educational supervision.

As academics debated the public's safety versus residents' educational requirements, University Hospital in Newark, the main teaching hospital for the University, served as the city's primary care provider. Through all portals every day, the city's residents stream in for care—trauma care, routine dental care, primary care, psychiatric care, obstetric care, oncology, and more. And, in the late 1980s, the intensity of care to those infected with the human immunodeficiency virus (HIV) was almost overwhelming. In fact, the sheer volume of HIV-positive patients mandated that a new care delivery system evolve in 1988. The Newark Autoimmune Deficiency Syndrome (AIDS) Consortium established the Broadway House for Continuing Care to manage the post-acute care needs for persons with AIDS. The complex morbidity of patients served at University Hospital was stunning. Charged by Stanley Bergen in 1986 to start nursing programs at the university, I was especially impressed with the urgency of acute care needs. The Newark Agreements, a document signed by local and state representatives in 1968 when the university was first established, had named the hospital as the city's primary care provider. It was very difficult to even begin to imagine primary care in the face of such disease, most prominently the rate of HIV-infected residents. So I began my career at UMDNJ, pregnant with my third child, charged to design nursing programs amidst the backdrop of exhausted medical residents, complex patients representing Newark's exceptionally poor population, and a real desire to help make it right.

Education of Nurse Practitioners

In late summer 1986, I interviewed for the position of chairperson, Department of Nursing Education and Services in the School of Health-Related Professions, on the Newark campus of the University of Medicine and Dentistry of New Jersey. The school was located in the old Martland Hospital building on Bergen Street. This fourteen-story hospital, with 750 beds, opened in 1958 and named after the revered Newark pathologist Dr. Harrison S. Martland. By 1979, this hospital was deemed obsolete, and a new hospital was built across the street. The Martland Hospital building, however, was retained and used for a variety of purposes once all patients and equipment were transported across the street. The school, including the Department of Nursing Education and Services, as well as various university administrative offices and out-patient services, relocated to Martland. The dean's suite was on the first floor, in the former offices of the hospital's chief executive officer. Nervous, and a bit nauseous (I was in the first trimester of my third pregnancy), I was fearful that I looked wilted by the heat, my hair falling flat down my neck, curls lost. My new dress seemed to have lost its crisp look in the late summer heat. Teresa Marsico, head of the school's Midwifery Program and a registered nurse, interviewed me for the position. She seemed leery of me. Why was I interested in the chair's position? In over a year, I was apparently the only candidate for the position. I found this intriguing; the interviewee became the interviewer. Teresa explained that many nurse leaders in the state did not support the establishment of nursing education programs at the university, the state's only academic health sciences institution. Fearful that medicine would subjugate nursing in a medically dominated hierarchy, academic nurse leaders stayed clear of the university. Stanley Bergen had closed the hospital's longstanding diploma school of nursing when

he arrived in 1970, and subsequently he created a joint associate degree nursing program with Essex County College—a program with poor passage rates of
graduates on the registered nurse licensing examination. Leaders focused on
baccalaureate nursing education were also not endeared to Bergen's choice of
partnership with an associate degree program.

Teresa's story seemed odd to me. Nursing, I was sure, was an integral part
of an academic health sciences university. Prior to accepting the position of
chair, I had been an assistant professor at Rutgers University College of Nursing, also located in Newark. In fact, these universities are part of Newark's University Heights, a section of the city housing Rutgers, UMDNJ, the New Jersey
Institute of Technology, and Essex County College. In my past Rutgers life, I
would drive down South Orange Avenue, passing University Hospital and all
the while marveling at the fact that UMDNJ did not have a nursing school of its
own. When offered the position, I quickly arranged my office in the Martland
Building to be as functional as possible. A long room, previously used as a
procedures room for in-patients, had a large stainless steel scrub sink with a
knee-action pedal and floor-to-ceiling light-green tiles. The tilt-latch window
was large, with years of grime clouding the outside. Given that the building
had been previously occupied, many of the fourteen floors had furniture long
abandoned but not yet discarded—a virtual mall of previously used office parts.
I retrofitted my office with a long table, several chairs of varying colors and
shapes, and pictures of my children. Calling my office motif Tupperware eclec-
tic, I was very satisfied with my new home, inclusive of an old, federal style
vintage steel desk.

I was also very satisfied being a part of the university team. While I held
a fairly new PhD in nursing, I was most proud of my credential as a certified critical care registered nurse, a member of the American Association of
Critical Care Nurses. My business cards included the CCRN credential after my
name, along with my academic credential. Knowing that my initial goal was
to close the failed joint venture with Essex County College, I did so quickly
in order to focus on designing future academic nursing programs to be offered
at the university. My background in critical care, against the backdrop of concerns over patient safety stimulated by residents' long hours of duty, led me
quickly to the nurse practitioner role. My hypothesis was simple: acute care
nurse practitioners would provide sustained in-patient hospitalist care to ill
clients, thus expanding care capacity. A pragmatist, I knew that the university
was not authorized to provide a four-year baccalaureate education, given its
charter as a health sciences university. However, it was chartered to provide
graduate education in the biomedical sciences; it was under this authority that

I designed a Master of Science in Nursing (MSN) degree program with an initial acute care nurse practitioner concentration. My five-year strategic plan mapped out the gradual phase-out of the associate degree program in 1988 and the establishment of an MSN program in 1990. Stanley Bergen accepted my plan, authorizing me to recruit faculty to design and implement the program, once it was operational.

While not a nurse practitioner, I was a critical care specialist. I turned to the National Organization of Nurse Practitioner Faculty for guidance on the curriculum. This organization, begun in 1974, has developed core competencies for nurse practitioners; these competencies have shaped national guidelines for nurse practitioner educational programs. The curriculum skeleton required basic sciences, including pathophysiology and clinical pharmacology, didactic and clinical education in the practice of acute advanced practice nursing care, and research and support courses related to the population served. Given the dearth of faculty in the department, the development of the curriculum was simple, almost recipe-like. A well-known nurse leader from the University of Texas Health Science Center School of Nursing at Houston, Dr. Patricia Starck, served as consultant for the program, giving guidance on accreditation standards and need for clinical resources. By 1988, a small team of nursing faculty—tenured and tenure-track—within the Department of Nursing Education and Services was prepared to undergo the state's Department of Higher Education and Board of Higher Education review and approval processes.

The curriculum had been designed with an intense last-semester internship in acute care practice—a three-day-per-week clinical practicum under the direct supervision of a clinical preceptor and a full-time nursing faculty member. This schedule was unique in graduate nursing education. In that the overwhelming majority of graduate nursing students are full-time employees and part-time students, most programs have evening classroom sessions and part-time clinical experiences. I felt quite passionate, however, that part-time engagement in acute care was inadequate if graduates were to provide hospitalist care in specialty services. Graduate nursing education, for the most part, caters to the needs of full-time employees—often, I feel, to the detriment of students' learning. Class during coffee break. While not, perhaps, that blatant, it is commonplace for nursing programs to be offered on-site at a health care facility to make it easier for students to attend classes. Even if our program had fewer enrollments, I held firm to my belief that clinical education required practice and validation of skills. Graduate internships are critical across health disciplines, including nursing as well as medicine and dentistry.

The program was therefore designed with advanced pharmacology and pathophysiology as core courses, with an emphasis on recognizing pathology via objective findings and subjective complaints. Knowledge of the clinical research literature, current therapies to manage diagnoses, and the critical reasoning skills to differentially diagnose patients' problems were all taught in separate graduate courses. Learning the practice of advanced acute care nursing requires time-at-task, under the watchful tutelage of seasoned clinicians. The program was designed so that students would first be taught how to conduct complete histories and physical examinations, and to determine possible causes of their chief complaints. They would learn to communicate therapeutically, to listen as patients told their stories; they would also be taught to assess the reliability of the narrator. Over four semesters, each sixteen weeks long, students would engage in progressively more complex patient management, culminating in a final immersion semester—or, internship. The program, once fully designed, was approved within the school and the university, and was subsequently forwarded to the New Jersey Department and Board of Higher Education for final review and endorsement.

Once the board and department received the university's document seeking approval for the graduate acute care nurse practitioner program in 1989, chaos ensued. Frankly, I couldn't believe that nurses across the state could galvanize their collective resources so quickly. Nurses in New Jersey receive the same registered nurse license, irrespective of education. This significant entry-into-practice issue—the scope of legal practice not based on educational attainment—was nursing's giant political gorilla lumbering in quiet aggression in an otherwise tranquil landscape. Clearly, the university's program threatened something that was core to the state's nursing community, a reality that I didn't truly appreciate at the onset. I thought the chaos was a skirmish, but it was really a full-fledged war against the university, which became a symbol for nursing's long-perceived wrongs imposed by medicine and hospital administration. I should not have been surprised; a key nursing leader had called me promising that I would never have another job in nursing in the state now that I had joined the medical university. I was a traitor, moving behind enemy lines.

On October 20, 1989, the New Jersey State Board of Higher Education held an all-day meeting to hear public testimony on the university's MSN program and to act on the application. The board's agenda for this meeting was a single item—approval of the MSN program. Normally, the agenda had multiple items and concluded in approximately two hours. For this single agenda item, however, the board had been deluged with comments, predominantly negative letters lobbied from the nursing community, including educators, New Jersey

State Nurses Association representatives, Board of Nursing members, and others. The meeting was held at Thomas Edison State College, located on West State Street in Trenton. Housed in one of Trenton's historic landmarks—the Kelsey Building, constructed in 1911—and offering adult distance-learning degree programs since 1972, the college provided an auspicious and regal backdrop for this potentially cantankerous event. Back at the university, Stanley Bergen directed this event with Academy Award–winning aplomb—a politically savvy statesman, with an amazing mix of arrogance and humility, packaged in a Lincolnesque comportment. For every opposing view, we researched a state or national figure to present a counterpoint view. All chits, all favors were called in. Colleagues from nursing, medicine and health administration, as well as potential patients, lined up to provide testimony. We rehearsed often, worrying over testimony style, content, appearance, tone, and order. I visited a colleague of Stanley Bergen—an administrator from a philanthropic foundation in New York—to advise me on my opening summary. Give them numbers, he demanded. He drilled me on data. People remember the last thing you say, he told me. Hit them with a number they won't forget.

I dressed carefully for this event. A light blue suit, with an A-line skirt and a light pink shirt with a high collar and navy floral neck tie. A university pin on my suit lapel. Confident that our cause was right and the ensuing chaos bizarre, I provided an opening summary of our application. Dr. Patricia Starck, the Department of Higher Education's consultant for our program, smiled calmly from her seat at the board's conference table. Light strawberry-colored hair, wearing a classic suit—a powerful presence cloaked in a diminutive frame. In her soft Texas drawl, Dr. Starck summarized her reasons for supporting the program. As she spoke, I recall thinking that rarely do traditional professions display such public acts of self-destruction. Classic professions manage their disagreements internally, presenting uniform public messages. Agreement to disagree. Opponents to the program presented a sanctimonious posture, somewhat reminiscent of nursing's religious beginnings. An aura of hypocritical piety—a tone difficult to defy, except with the reality of numbers. At the conclusion of my opening summary, I noted that New Jersey had among the lowest passage rates for graduates taking the registered nurse licensing examination and that our state was notorious for being one of the last states to legislate nurse practitioners as care providers. *Let me say that again*, I concluded, by repeating my statement and calling for change. In all future campaigns to change behavior, I have focused concluding statements on numbers—concrete data universally understood, providing successful messages.

The dean for our School of Osteopathic Medicine provided our lead testimony, after which testimony was heard from alternating sides. The left side—the groom's side—housed the university community, the male side representing academic medicine and hospital administration. The right side—the bride's side—included all those from the nursing community opposing the approval of the acute care nurse practitioner program. Sensitive to the intense passions evoked by this program, Chancellor T. Edward Hollander charged the board to consider the following question as they reviewed the university's application: Will the program contribute to the enhancement of patient care by advancing the professional competence of practicing nurses and offering greater upward mobility for nurses?

Ninety people testified during that hearing, equally matched in favor or opposition. Claiming that the university was creating a new type of nurse requiring investigation by the New Jersey State Board of Nursing, the board's president reported that she needed to examine the practice implications of a "new" nurse in New Jersey. In fact, a 1989 paper—"Nurses United for the Public Good"—circulated throughout the room during the session. Signed by nurse leaders—including presidents of the New Jersey State Nurses Association, New Jersey League for Nursing, the New Jersey Association of Baccalaureate and Higher Degree Nursing Programs, the Organization of Nurse Executives/New Jersey, the New Jersey Council of Associate Degree Nursing Programs, and the Association of Diploma Schools of Professional Nursing—and addressed to President Deborah Wolfe, this paper indicated that the acute care nurse practitioner program lacked documented need and was an unwise use of tax dollars. I was nonplussed by nursing's fear of oppression at the hands of Stanley Bergen, president of UMDNJ. He symbolized a wicked past and a frightful future. Living in the interstices between these groups, I was liberated to try new ideas· and to amass a group of nursing faculty willing to live on the fringe. Once on the fringe, I fully expected disapproval from the nursing community; I also anticipated a strong applicant pool to our programs endorsed nationally but dismissed locally.

Opponents to the program testified with emotional fervor, accusing the university of intending to prepare little doctors. Registered nurses employed at University Hospital testified against their employer. As in the Disney movie, lemmings ran to the sea. New Jersey nurses opposed the program, nurses from other states supported it. A most prominent opponent was Rutgers—the State University of New Jersey College of Nursing, also located in Newark, within a few miles from the University of Medicine and Dentistry of New Jersey. Rutgers had enjoyed a strong relationship with the nursing department at University

Hospital and vehemently opposed any competition to this relationship, one that provided them full reign over the hospital's clinical services and continuing education opportunities. Rutgers also offered graduate nursing programs, the essential provider of public nursing education in northern New Jersey.

At the conclusion of all testimony, Dr. Deborah T. Wolfe, the president of the board, proclaimed *Alleluia! This has been a great day!* Pleased that all voices had been heard, President Wolfe and the board sought compromise in its final action. The board required that the University of Medicine and Dentistry of New Jersey and Rutgers University attempt to accomplish the goals of the new acute care nurse practitioner program within the existing Rutgers master's degree program; and only if this collaborative effect could not be realized would UMDNJ be empowered to proceed with the implementation of the MSN program. After months of negotiation with Rutgers officials and nursing faculty members, talks failed, compromise unable to be reached. On March 23, 1990, the acute care nurse practitioner program moved into full planning, with intent to bring a first class of students on the health science campus in fall 1990. The negotiations were tense between the two opponents: the Rutgers team, with 224 years of classic strength behind it, and the UMDNJ team, a young upstart academic health sciences university evolving from the Newark riots of 1967. Being young, however, we were able to say no more easily than our opponents. We were quite open in our comments; at one meeting I indicated that my teeth hurt with the sweetness of their words! One senior official at UMDNJ reminded me often that our small team of three nursing faculty members at that negotiation table had real power—one with a foot on the gas pedal, one on the brake, and one gripping the steering wheel. As claimed by writer Joan Whitlow in the *Newark Star-Ledger* (October 21, 1989), the drama between UMDNJ and Rutgers was a turf fight.

In fall 1990, our acute care nurse practitioner program was implemented. Paralleling this program, however, was an equally arduous and unexpected challenge. Concurrent with our plans for establishing the nurse practitioner program, we had also planned—consistent with my original strategic plan designed in 1986—a joint Associate of Science in Nursing program with Middlesex County College, to begin in fall 1990. Middlesex County College had a long and successful history in associate degree nursing education. Over time, however, its graduates' passage rates on the registered nurse licensing examination had declined, and the college's reputation was put at stake, with a largely tenured nursing faculty unwilling to significantly change its methods or curriculum. Joining with the university, the college would continue to offer a nursing program, but the locus of control for the nursing faculty would emanate from the university, with a faculty fully engaged in a practice plan, remaining current with practice requirements.

The acute care nurse practitioner program and the associate degree program inevitably became interwoven as anathema to the nursing community. A group called the Coalition of Concerned Nurses (CCN) worked arduously to destroy all of the university's nursing initiatives, from the associate degree program to the graduate program to the very idea of an eventual school of nursing to house these programs. CCN—an entity incorporated by a nurse leader who at different times was the executive to the New Jersey State Nurses Association and an assemblywoman in the state legislature. We faced a wall of solid opposition. Nurse leaders voiced disbelief that UMDNJ had the statutory authority to offer nursing, given that it was legislated to offer biomedical degrees. The New Jersey State Nurses Association worried if academic nursing programs were offered at UMDNJ, would nursing go back under medical control?

The Board of Nursing, as well as the Board of Higher Education, approved the joint Associate of Science in Nursing program in spring 1990. The Coalition of Concerned Nurses filed a legal case against the Board of Nursing, UMDNJ, the Board of Higher Education, and the Department of Higher Education in summer 1990. On July 16, 1990, the Appellate Division of the Superior Court of New Jersey heard the coalition's case that the university did not have the statutory authority to confer an associate of science degree with a major in nursing. A panel of three judges concluded in favor of the university (Superior Court of New Jersey, Appellate Division, Argued July 16, 1990; Decided July 31, 1990). The judges held that UMDNJ was authorized to provide undergraduate nursing education programs through joint efforts with two-and four-year colleges and general university campuses in the state. When one judge asked a representative of the coalition *What is the real problem here?* the representative said that *everyone knows that men run women at UMDNJ.* Without blinking, the judge responded that *the court could not solve such psychological issues.*

But the battle didn't end at that point and has not ended still. Were it not for a tradition of legislation, nursing would never have realized any gains beyond those associated with virtue.

Chapter 4

Protection of the Public
or Creation of a Guild?

Helmets down, lancets up! According to a colleague, here is an apt motto for nursing, complete with medieval associations. Experiences with boards of nursing hardened me to nursing's own brand of inquisition. A national model—termed LACE (Licensure, Accreditation, Credentialing, and Education)—emerged in 2008 in an effort to unify and standardize requirements for nurse practitioner practice across states. Despite the emergence of this model, however, self-oppression continues, just as social philosopher Michel Foucault hypothesized. Unique forms of discipline include special rules by boards of nursing, aimed at compliance or subsequent punishment, to dictate clinical education ratios of faculty to students, circumscribe curricula, specify faculty requirements, and define program resources with no regard to institutional context. Even as nursing's so-called bone and sinew, the registered nurse, practices under a single license that denies scope of practice based on educational levels, nurse administrators with advanced education remorselessly advocate for diploma-prepared nursing workforces. Here is a nightmare in which workforce needs trump the value of education and the future of the individual. Yet even as nursing's subtle mistrust of its own plays out in mandates, individuals move hopefully forward, championing special causes. My experiences with school-based wellness centers illustrate such advocacy. Anticipating correctly the Supreme Court's 2012 endorsement of the Patient Protection and Affordable Care Act, my Philadelphia nursing colleagues established nurse practitioner school-based clinics at two charter schools in 2010–2011. With nurse practitioners in place,

the absenteeism rate plummeted at the end of year one, heralding the value of the effort and forecasting success of some components of the health care reform law. Hardiness is necessary but not sufficient to buffet nursing's own culture; resilience coupled with hopefulness for future change is also required. The story of Joe at Mary Howard Health Center highlights this resilience. One patient–one provider haughtiness takes time to cultivate.

*

Head down against the wind, a dark brown woolen scarf wrapped tightly around her neck, Irene Fallon marched confidently on the icy street toward Newark City Hospital in Newark on December 4, 1901. Set against the crisp, deep blue evening sky, the hospital was a formidable four-story red brick structure, first occupied in 1890. The bright golden bells hanging from the large pine Christmas wreath on the main hospital door jingled loudly as Irene entered the building. A young graduate of the Cooper Hospital Training School for Nurses in Camden, Irene walked briskly to the nurses' quarters. Nurses had gathered in the large, impeccably clean and scantily furnished main hall, seated comfortably around a large spruce tree, decorated with strings of popcorn and homemade ornaments. Excitement and anticipation were in the air. The nurses' goal, as noted in the minutes of that meeting: to organize the New Jersey State Nurses Association for the purpose of securing legislation that would lead to the betterment of the nursing profession. Efforts of this New Jersey group were watched vigilantly by members of the Nurses Associated Alumnae of the United States and Canada, created in 1897 with three goals, as documented by Susan Reverby in *Annual Conventions, 1893–1899: The American Society of Superintendents of Training Schools for Nurses* (1985): to establish and maintain a code of ethics, to elevate the standard of nursing education, and to promote the usefulness, honor, and the financial and other interests of nursing. Like its colleague organization, the American Society of Superintendents of Training Schools for Nurses, the alumnae association germinated in the period surrounding the 1893 Chicago World's Fair, a period when teachers, engineers, and others crafted professional identities through organizational structure and shared goals. The date marked the entrance of the United States as a leader within the international community.

By the end of that December evening, Irene had been elected president of the new state organization by its 112 charter members. Her first charge as president was to secure state registration of nurses, an action considered tantamount to self-preservation, eliminating unqualified quacks from practicing the profession. Lobbying tenaciously, Irene and her fellow officers of the NJSNA secured friends in the legislature, galvanizing positive votes for the Nursing Practice law. In April 1903, the act to license graduate nurses was signed into law by Republican governor Franklin Murphy (Chapter 109, *Laws of New Jersey*, 1903). To receive a license from a county clerk, an applicant had to present a diploma from a training school for nurses offered by a hospital that required at least two years of practical and classroom training—plus a fifty-cent fee. Success. The registered nurse license—the RN—would now signify authenticity, title protection by law, and professionalization through law rather than education, the standard route open to other disciplines.

More than one hundred years later, legislation remains the vehicle for continued advancement in nursing. As other professions evolved through higher education, nursing remained tethered to hospitals and to medicine, incrementally expanding its scope of practice through amendments to nurse practice laws.

Local Rule, Local Power

By 2012, the term Advanced Practice Registered Nurse (APRN) had been widely adopted by nurse leaders and educators throughout the country to identify those who provide direct care to individuals. This acronym—APRN—was embedded in a 2008 document entitled *Consensus Model for APRN Regulation: Licensure, Accreditation, Certification, and Education.* Multiple professional nursing groups—in fact, forty-six organizations—participated in generating this consensus model, which proposed to align the licensure, accreditation, certification, and education (LACE) of APRNs to improve patient safety and expand access to these providers.

This model remains a goal. Since state boards of nursing were first established in the early twentieth century, they did so without conforming to a national model or to commonly accepted national standards. Each state's Board of Nursing reserves the right to independently determine the APRN's legal scope of practice, roles recognized, eligibility criteria for practice, and certification examinations approved to ascertain competency as an entry-level APRN. This diversity in licensing APRNs across states presents interesting barriers to nurse practitioners who wish to travel between and among states.

In leaving New Jersey to accept a position at Temple University in Pennsylvania, I felt that I had opened a Pandora's box of barriers to practice nursing. In fact, for a short time I worried that I would be in the interesting position of chair of a nursing department, but unlicensed to practice in that state. Once I

had accepted the position at Temple University, I immediately turned my attention to obtaining my registered nurse license and my certification to practice as
a nurse practitioner in Pennsylvania. Obtaining my RN license by endorsement
was not difficult. However, the process to receive certification as an Adult NP
in Pennsylvania was challenging. Submission of transcripts of my undergraduate education as well as all graduate education did not suffice; additionally, I
needed to forward syllabi of courses I had taken in my nurse practitioner program. Fortunately, I knew people at the university who could locate these syllabi for me. Even these, however, were not enough to verify that I had clinical
pharmacology, pathophysiology, or primary care content required for certification. Eventually, I requested the dean of the UMDNJ School of Nursing to verify
my educational background for the Pennsylvania board. I am tenacious and
fairly well connected—even with this, the delays were stunning. Acceptance of
my transcripts from fully accredited institutions did not suffice as verification
of my legitimacy. More was demanded. As I went through this process, I put
my blinders on and plowed ahead, feeling somewhat like the tired horses that
trudge around Central Park in Manhattan, carrying sightseers around at holiday
season to be scandalized by Bergdorf Goodman's windows. I never questioned
the demands. Retribution always follows sin, and questioning a bureaucracy is
surely sinful.

The Pennsylvania State Board of Nursing also requires that all nursing faculty be approved by that agency, prior to serving in the role. The Nursing Faculty
Qualifications Form includes sections on academic qualifications, licensure and
certification information, and professional qualifications. Not a user-friendly
form, it must be downloaded and typed, then submitted with any necessary
additional documentation. After a lengthy conversation with an administrator
at the board, I forwarded my form in early September 2008. In spring 2009 I
received a letter from the board approving my role as chair of the department,
months after the Temple board of trustees had appointed me as a tenured professor to the administrative role of chair. Surely approving an individual to serve
as administrator in a college and university was outside the scope of the board's
purview, I thought. Again, however, I retained my letter, showing it only to a
certain few for gallows humor.

My humor about this foolishness cloaked my fears and embarrassment
about the board's actions. Evident was their excessive need to control the very
professionals they regulate, a pervasive lack of trust permeating all aspects of
the board's actions. While my experiences with the New Jersey State Board of
Nursing relative to approval of new undergraduate prelicensure programs was
fraught with challenges, I understood those challenges to be flavored by the

board's mistrust of my university president—a physician—and his seemingly voracious appetite to control health care delivery in the state. If I had been an outsider looking in at the university, I would almost have understood the New Jersey board's reticence in trusting my president, especially in the context of nursing's growth as a discipline in the United States. The New Jersey board, however, did not seek to approve my appointment to the university, nor did it establish criteria for approval of nurse practitioner educational programs. Once settled in at Temple, the difference between the functions of the two state boards began to fascinate me.

Approval and Accreditation

Early in my first fall 2008 semester at Temple University, a graduate program faculty member asked to meet with me. *Do you know the Pennsylvania Board of Nursing requirements for the number of students a faculty member can supervise clinically?* she asked. I knew it was a trick question. While I had not yet digested Title 49, Professional and Vocational Standards, of the Pennsylvania Code, I was up to speed on the number of students the program director had assigned to each faculty member. I assured her that I knew this information. She suddenly waved a page photcopied from the board's regulations at me, her voice becoming louder and her tone shrill. *Six*, she said, *only six! And I have more than six in my group!* Her face became blotchy red, and her hands shook. She was in a rage. The clinical courses in the Master of Science in Nursing (MSN) program at Temple operated similarly to the majority of such programs—each student in a clinical course is assigned a preceptor to directly mentor the student. One faculty member is assigned to make site visits to each student-preceptor pair throughout a semester to provide guidance, support, and evaluation. Clinical preceptors are nurse practitioners or physicians who agree to assume this role and who understand the course requirements and intended outcomes.

My colleague faculty administrator and I were in an interesting situation. In her zeal, she had aggressively marketed the program, resulting in what every university wants—an increase in enrollment. Our faculty ranks, however, did not increase proportionately. Our faculty did indeed have a few more than six students in each clinical course. Even as we sought new faculty lines, I knew that it would take time for such a request to be reviewed, and if possible, honored. In the meantime, as the demand for primary care providers for inner cities increased, I refused to drop enrollment simply due to what I considered a spurious board regulation. I thought that a reasonable approach was simply to discuss this requirement with board members; this conversation became increasingly important when my faculty member reported me to the board as noncompliant.

The genesis of the 1 faculty to 6 students (1:6) ratio in a clinical course derives from guidelines published by the National Organization of Nurse Practitioner Faculty (NONPF). A voluntary organization, NONPF also recommends that the faculty/student ratio for direct supervision is 1:2 if faculty members are not seeing their own patients and 1:1 if faculty are seeing their own patients. These three recommendations for faculty/student ratios were adopted by the Pennsylvania State Board of Nursing. These ratios provide a rate-limiting control on the annual graduation rate of nurse practitioners; thus, they also curb the capacity of colleges and universities to infuse the state with additional primary care providers. In my phone conference with representatives from the board, I asked if these board requirements were strictly enforced, wondering aloud about the magnitude of my competitors personnel budgets. The response was vague. I was told that the board looks at the whole picture, and the conversation terminated.

Our MSN program continued with a noncompliant faculty-to-student ratio. In a spring 2009 meeting, my angry faculty member pointed her finger at me and announced passionately that *This is* not *New Jersey!* Our agenda topic was approval of new graduate-level courses that would eventually be part of a Doctor of Nursing Practice (DNP) program. She was simply reminding me that the Board of Nursing in New Jersey—as compared to Pennsylvania's board— does not mandate any requirements for nurse practitioner programs, preferring instead to accept certification from an accredited national certification organization. She was correct; Pennsylvania is a highly regulated state. And, given that we planned to transition our MSN program to a DNP program format effective fall 2010, I knew that I needed to visit with board representatives to review the requirements for approval of a new nurse practitioner program.

Special Rules, Aimed at Compliance

At an early hour on a May morning in 2009, I left my home in southern New Jersey for an excursion to the Pennsylvania State Board of Nursing in Harrisburg. My goal was a simple one—to find out exactly how to compose my application seeking approval to transition from a Master of Science in Nursing (MSN) nurse practitioner program to a Doctor of Nursing Practice (DNP) nurse practitioner program. Our transition from an MSN to a DNP program was prompted by action of the American Association of Colleges of Nursing. The move to a DNP degree—a clinical doctorate—is consistent with a growing trend for health care providers to award such degrees, somewhat on the heels of a 2003 Institute of

Medicine report entitled *Health Professions Education: A Bridge to Quality.* This report fueled change among health professions' doctoral degrees.

My visit to the Board of Nursing was critical: I wanted to write the required document right the first time. I had a meeting planned with two nursing practice advisors of the board. Both were fully versed in the details outlined in sections 21.361 through 21.377: *Approval of Certified Registered Nurse Practitioner Programs* of Title 49 of the Pennsylvania Code. These sections required responses on questions involving organizational structure, faculty qualifications, curriculum content, evaluation methods, facility and resource requirements, selection and admission standards, and program records. The details demanded were daunting. The information required, for example, documentation of advanced pharmacology content in the curriculum, including details on drug categories to be taught, drug pharmacodynamics, drug pharmacotherapeutics, patient education to be provided, legal requirements, safety aspects of prescribing, and more. The section on pharmacology alone entailed a laundry list of medications—categories, prototypes, routes of administration, and so forth. Time was critical. In order to accept students into our new program in fall 2010, we needed to achieve approvals from three groups, including first the college and then the university, and the Pennsylvania Board of Nursing.

So I drove to Harrisburg, a three and a half-hour drive from my home. As it turned out, my colleague at Temple who had planned to come did not join me. So I journeyed alone to visit the nursing practice advisors at the board. It was a beautiful day, with most of my ride on the Pennsylvania Turnpike, Route 76 West. With the luxury of driving alone, I saw the pastoral state truly for the first time. Beautiful, rolling fields of corn and other produce, with farm equipment, bales of hay, and horses and goats roaming contentedly without noticing one another. The quiet beauty of Pennsylvania charmed, and calmed, me. As I drove off the exit ramp 247 on Route 76, I realized that I was now in the state's capital, Harrisburg: low-lying buildings, with space and trees and scrubs between them, and parking on the street. At one point, on a local road, I stopped at a light. At my left was an Amish family in a traditional buggy, with large round spoked wheels and a covered carriage compartment, connected to a young, strong chestnut-brown horse. The driver nodded to me, tipping the rim of his broad-brimmed hat. At his side was a young woman, her hair drawn back into a classic Amish white headpiece, with sashes draped neatly over her shoulders. Her head remained bowed. I turned my radio down, the music of Sting sounding sacrilegious in their presence. Not quite like my previous experiences in Newark and Camden. Absolutely lovely.

The Board of Nursing is located within a three-story building in the center of the city. The building, not immediately recognizable as a state entity, felt warm. The receptionist in the main hall directed me to the nursing section, waving and encouraging me to *have a nice day*. I was ushered into a large rectangular-shaped conference room, filled with the musty aroma of old paper, anchored by a table capable of seating at least twenty people. I was asked to take a seat at one end of the table. As I settled in and placed my unruly pens, papers, and regulatory books on my area of the table, my two nursing practice advisor colleagues entered the room. Formal, stately. I explained Temple's goal to transition the existing MSN nurse practitioner program to the DNP format.

The Temple nursing faculty was eager to have their DNP program approved. A DNP degree prepares registered nurses with baccalaureate degrees to become certified as advanced practice nurses. Once certified by a professional nursing organization, DNP graduates can then become licensed by their state Board of Nursing as advanced practice nurses, with a scope of practice defined by regulation. The DNP is a nursing degree; the certification to practice is awarded by boards of nursing. The Medical Doctor (MD) degree prepares baccalaureate graduates to sit for licensure by state boards of medicine or boards of medical examiners for the MD license, with a scope of practice defined by medical regulations. A wide area of commonality between the MD and DNP licenses is that of primary care practice, with both groups—one defined by medical regulations and the other by nursing regulations—diagnosing and managing common acute and chronic health problems of individuals. Transitioning from the MSN degree to the DNP degree would be a major accomplishment for the faculty. Their pride was on the table, along with my pens.

With the goal for the meeting established we then reviewed, page by page, the documentation required to obtain approval of our new program. It would not be considered an amended program, but rather a completely new program. In fact, since we sought to transition two MSN program tracks—the adult nurse practitioner track and the family nurse practitioner track—to the DNP format, the advisors informed me that two approval documents needed to be submitted. Despite the fact that these two tracks differed only by one course, two complete documents were required. Paper documents, double-spaced, single-sided, one-inch margins, size 12-point font. Seventeen copies of each, held together with large bull clips. The digital world was as remote there as it would be on the Amish farms. Line-by-line, we reviewed the Board of Nursing regulations for approval of certified registered nurse practitioner programs. No reprieve would be possible. The nauseating detail of these documents would kill the best of women; but I had been steeled by past experiences with the New Jersey

Board of Nursing through the startup of two baccalaureate programs. I could do this in the summer, or so I thought.

I fought back my anger as I sat at the table. My dispassionate external demeanor remained flat as I struggled to scream *this is crazy!* Be calm. In the fast-paced world of electronic medical records, e-learning paperless courses, and our knowledge of the global burden of disease, I would ultimately produce two documents over nine months with five drafts, each final copy approximately four hundred pages and copied seventeen times. Slow down, relinquish control, submit obediently, prove your worthiness, and survive predator, dronelike demands of insentient bureaucrats.

Upon completion of my post-master's certificate program as an adult nurse practitioner at the University of Medicine and Dentistry of New Jersey in 1998, I sat for both the American Academy of Nurse Practitioners (AANP) and the American Nurses Credentialing Center (ANCC) certification examinations. I then submitted my application for certification as an adult nurse practitioner as outlined by the Board of Nursing. This process included documentation that I was a licensed registered nurse in the state, that I had graduated from an accredited nurse practitioner educational program, and that I held certification as an adult nurse practitioner through either the AANP or the ANCC. I received my original adult nurse practitioner certification from the New Jersey Board of Nursing in 1998; I framed the certificate, a document that I was extremely proud of earning. The process was straightforward. This state board deferred to criteria promulgated by professional organizations to assure that candidates for certification had been appropriately educated to provide safe care to the public—a voluntary, peer process. Sitting at the long table at the headquarters of the Pennsylvania State Board of Nursing, I wondered if I was still dealing with the same profession.

Invisible Victory

After ten months and five drafts of applications to the Pennsylvania State Board of Nursing seeking approval of two Doctor of Nursing Practice (DNP) programs—one for an Adult Nurse Practitioner program and the second for a Family Nurse Practitioner program—we were on the Board's April 13, 2010, agenda as action items. The board rotates its business meetings across the state, and on this day in April the meeting was held at Villanova University College of Nursing.

It was a grim day, the atmosphere heavy with rain and fast-moving, dull gray clouds. The sidewalks were wet, puddles everywhere, with yellow bell-shaped blooms of forsythia bushes lining the major roads in Villanova,

Pennsylvania—early evidence of springtime to come. I was guardedly excited about the meeting. Joining me was one of my nursing colleagues, an experienced, longtime member of Temple University and well known in the Philadelphia nursing community. As the administrator directly responsible for supervision of the nurse practitioner programs, she needed to be present at this meeting. Though an experienced nurse educator, she was not a certified nurse practitioner. When joining Temple, I had argued with the Board of Nursing to retain her in her role, given that she had served successfully in that role prior to my employment. The board begrudgingly approved her appointment as director of the nurse practitioner program, solely on the basis that she reported to me. I was taken by the board's dismissive attitude about the individual's administrative talent. I had experienced something similar to this while an administrator in New Jersey. I had recommended that a master's-prepared nurse be named the assistant dean for our Stratford, southern New Jersey, campus. A formidable administrator previously responsible for a medical center's surgical service, she was exactly the practical, detailed person I needed to establish a branch campus. The university's Board of Trustees, however, questioned naming someone to this position who did not hold an earned doctoral degree. Again, with begrudging approval, the board did name my candidate as the assistant dean, but only after my arguments that her talents in administration were more relevant to what was needed than her level of education. To the present day, I am exasperated by the lack of respect afforded administrative talent as essential to the smooth operation of a unit, irrespective of that unit's mission or goals.

My colleague, a fan of her accelerator, had virtually flown us that day to Villanova University. We arrived in record time, my nerves a bit rattled and my mind racing to find a safe alternative to get a ride back to Temple when the meeting was convened. The meeting was scheduled in the auditorium of Driscoll Hall, a $32 million, state-of-the-art structure completed in July 2008. Certified as a green building by the U.S. Green Building Council, Driscoll Hall is a 75,500 square-foot building close to the main gate and adjacent to the Health Sciences Building that contains classrooms, seminar rooms, a simulation center, a center for nursing research and scholarship, a history of nursing room, a room for prayer and reflection, offices, and other areas for faculty, students, staff, and visitors. Stonemasonry, brick, and wood surrounded by grass and shrubs—an elegant structure in a peaceful green environment that elicited deep envy from the Philadelphia visitors. Our nursing department at Temple University is housed in the College of Health Professions and Social Work, in a building that was formerly the residence hall for students of the hospital's past diploma school of nursing—Jones Hall. Jones Hall, a ten-story dormitory structure reminiscent of the modern era's characteristic functionality, housed several departments within the college as well as administrative offices for the university. While this 1962 building was exclusively nursing's in its heyday, nursing was now squeezed into one floor with additional office space on a second floor. We clearly came from a different part of Philadelphia, the poor northern section of the city. Our mission, goals, and aspirations were reflections of our inner-city urban neighborhoods. While our confidence remained intact about the quality of our DNP program, we were certainly humbled by the grand edifice of our host university. Money can intercept a level playing field.

We parked in an area under construction, with mud and construction debris scattered across the lot. Walking precariously from one chunk of debris to another, feeling foolish as my umbrella turned inside out, we arrived wind-blown at the doors of Driscoll Hall well in advance of the meeting time. Recovering our composure with lipstick and brushing through dank hair, we found seats in the center area of the auditorium, just a few rows from the stage. The room smelled new, without any student graffiti on desks, backs of chairs, or walls. The room, indeed the building, contained religious symbols on walls, again quite unlike those in my own secular world. The building demanded reverence and respect. For me, there, I felt far above my own daily life, as if I could somehow control my life without actually living in it. Crucifixes suspend animation. My life on the streets of Newark, Camden, and North Philadelphia was distant as I tried to place my books and other papers neatly on the floor in front of me, without causing undue noise. I felt clumsy.

Early in my nursing education career, I had taught for a brief period at Seton Hall University in South Orange, New Jersey. Seton Hall, also a Catholic institution, had an ambiance not unlike Villanova's, with religious symbols, crucifixes, and other icons clearly visible. I have historically found it difficult to reconcile the religious tenets influencing nursing curricula with the practical health realities of urban life. I found myself daydreaming about the sheer volume of condoms I liberally distribute at the Mary Howard Health Center. How would my family-planning practices be viewed at both Villanova and Seton Hall? Pregnancy prevention—outside of sexual abstinence—would not be taught in these nursing programs. Family planning, stonemasonry, and forsythia blended together. I was anxious for the meeting to conclude.

The Pennsylvania State Board of Nursing consists of thirteen members. This includes a commissioner of Professional and Occupational Affairs, three public members, six registered nurses with at least three of these holding master's degrees in nursing, two licensed practical nurses, and one licensed dietitian-nutritionist. The chairperson of the board was a well-known, respected nurse practitioner and academic clinician, someone I believed would be a very appropriate peer to review our application documents. The board, however, relied on the evaluation and recommendation of a professional staff member. For the nine-month gestation leading up to this meeting, this advisor provided feedback on my documents, taking each line in the regulations as a mandate to document, quite without regard for redundancy or flow. I felt like I was in the middle of a major bean-counting contest, yet strangely supported by this advisor, who worked closely with me to make sure that the final product would be acceptable to the board. I complied with her suggestions. It was her summary recommendation document to the board that was important. I dared not offend, fearful of retribution. She provided a verbal summation to the board, and my colleague and I answered the questions that arose. The questions were minor, seemingly almost forced, just to ensure that some questions were raised. One public member wanted assurances that our funding would be sustained; we answered affirmatively. The members voted unanimously to approve our two new programs, and after handshakes and smiles, we drove off to an International House of Pancakes to celebrate.

At IHOP, we were met by our colleague, the undergraduate program administrator, who kindly congratulated us with effusive compliments. A small-framed, highly energetic administrator with an effervescent personality, she gave us the positive accolades we so badly needed to hear. Her cheery mood, however, could not impact our flat affect. We were relieved but quiet, knowing that our small department had a major transition ahead of us. Resource-poor—we had neither a departmental secretary nor an extensive simulation laboratory—and very busy, we had little time to celebrate. When I e-mailed my dean about our board approvals, his sole response was *wow*. The significance of offering a clinical primary care doctoral program seemed to elude him, as did an understanding of the term "primary care." As often happens, the daily busy—as my older daughter refers to the work that must be completed each work day—overwhelms, preventing time spent on issues that are perhaps of greater importance.

A twelve-panel board acted on a primary care nurse practitioner program, including three certified registered nurse practitioners, three public members, three licensed practical nurses, one registered nurse, one certified registered nurse anesthetist, and the deputy secretary/ commissioner for Regulatory Programs members. This composition was skewed: the number of members whose expertise in evaluating the program applications was inadequate; and the possibility of a negative vote in a board with six non-nurses and six nurses, and of the latter six, only three certified registered nurse practitioners. The push for consumerism and accountability, championed in the 1960s by lawyer Ralph Nader, led to the uncertainty that boards of health professions were capable of self-regulation, as explored in the U.S. Department of Health, Education, and Welfare's 1971 report *Report on Licensure and Related Health Personnel.*

Credentialing

With a victory behind us, we said goodbye in IHOP's parking lot.

New Jersey's and Pennsylvania's Boards of Nursing were challenging, but in different ways. In New Jersey, my challenges were political. Being part of a health sciences university with a physician as president, organized nursing—indeed, the Coalition of Concerned Nurses, representing the majority of professional organizations and academic programs in the state—viciously attacked me and others within the institution as traitors to the profession. I was perceived to have aligned with the enemy—medicine, our notorious oppressor. After the initial shock of personal attacks passed (one nurse leader had told me that she understood that I must have felt physically safe at the medical university, given that I had experienced a stroke with the birth of my third child, and thus proximity to medical care must have been important to me—the construing of rationale to explain my aberrant behavior), the political challenges in New Jersey were surprisingly liberating to me. I could be unrestrained in my thinking, freed from nursing's intellectual narrowness—the training wheels had been removed. The New Jersey battle, interestingly, was managed with a strategic plan replete with objective data.

In Pennsylvania, almost two decades later, my challenges in establishing a DNP program for nurse practitioners were more private, almost solitary. From July 2009 through April 2010, my relationship with the nursing practice advisor at the Board of Nursing was reminiscent of my work at New York University with my doctoral dissertation chair. Multiple drafts of two documents were submitted. Phone calls and e-mails from her struck terror in my soul, requiring Lamaze breathing exercises prior to responding. Reengaging my Catholic school obedience, I eventually responded compliantly. I felt trapped by this process. To veer independently into a new academic direction, to document a program designed to meet evolving health care challenges, was forbidden—and could jeopardize the programs' approval. It was a very private enterprise. At our faculty meetings, I reported that I continued to work with our Board of Nursing on approval of the programs. Outside of a cursory look by our graduate program administrator—who laughed understandingly—and a brief review of budgetary processes by an assistant dean at the college level, the process belonged to me. It was dreadfully depleting.

Different landscapes in Pennsylvania and in the Garden State. In New Jersey, I fenced with nursing's demons of external oppression—the gendered fear that medicine would control the profession. In Pennsylvania, I was forced to manage something more frightening, more cruel—nursing's oppression of itself, oppression metaphorically expressed by Michel Foucault's internal, complicit panopticism.

Cognitive Protoplasm

In joining Temple in summer 2008, I thought it odd that a state-supported public research university located in Philadelphia would offer diploma nursing programs under its aegis. Under the Temple University Health System, two affiliated hospitals ran diploma nursing programs—one at Episcopal Hospital and the second at Northeastern Hospital, both community hospitals in northern Philadelphia. Given my experience in New Jersey of helping the Englewood Hospital Diploma School of Nursing transition to a baccalaureate-degree-granting institution in cooperation with Ramapo College of New Jersey and the University of Medicine and Dentistry of New Jersey, I met with the chief nurse executive of the health system to explore a similar transition for the two diploma programs under the Temple umbrella. We subsequently met with my dean, the associate dean for academic affairs, and the health system's president and chief executive officer. We met in the dental school conference room. This room, located on the third floor of the Kornberg Dental School—referred to by locals, of course, as the "cornball" school—is past the school's museum of historic dental artifacts, including old dental chairs, equipment reminiscent of the *Little Shop of Horrors*, and various dental prostheses, a charming exhibit that must be reckoned with when exiting the elevator. How can an entire building smell like a dentist's office? The aromas were pleasant to me, since I so admired my own dentist in New Jersey, an African American man who floated jazz music through his entire dental suite. I had learned much from him about being a health care provider. His gentle speech, his ability to hide from plain sight the instruments that were on display in the Kornberg school, and respect for his dental team were admirable. While I was OK in that third-floor corridor—jazz entering my consciousness—my colleagues were not as pleased with the smells and their recollections of personal dentistry. We were ushered into a large office with a leather couch, leather chairs, and a large wooden desk, impressive to me for its lack of papers and other signs of current activity. I sank into a corner of the couch. It had a faint smell of leather, always symbolic of wealth—my conference room contained Tupperware chairs. My dean came from behind the desk, sitting in one of the chairs; the health system president sat in the other chair. We three women—the associate dean, also a nurse, the chief nurse executive, and I—sat on the couch. I was in kindergarten with the teachers looming before me.

We had a lively discussion. We explored the genesis of diploma schools of nursing, their links to hospitals, the history of nursing students providing all of the nursing care delivered in hospitals, and the gradual movement of nursing into higher education. I was thrilled; the two men—the dean and the health system president—listened attentively. Conceptually, by the end of our almost two-hour meeting, the group agreed that transitioning the health system's two diploma programs to a baccalaureate framework was appropriate for a university. As we gathered our belongings in readiness to exit, my mind racing on to the next steps, the president (and CEO) of the health system called me back for advice. He said that he wanted to start a nursing school at a third hospital within the health system, Jeanes Hospital, since he needed a nursing workforce. A stunning request, given the context.

The high-minded previous discussion had nothing whatsoever to do with workforce demands. Coming at the beginning of my tenure at Temple University, this meeting became the symbol of nursing's place within the health care context in Pennsylvania. In 2010, the National League for Nursing Accreditation Commission indicated that it accredited fifty-four diploma schools throughout the county. Of these fifty-four accredited programs, twenty (37%) are located in Pennsylvania. Pennsylvania offers more diploma nursing education programs than any other state. In fact, New Jersey, with ten schools (or 18.5%), comes in second. The remaining twenty-four programs are located in fourteen states, with the majority of states (thirty-four, or 68%) no longer offering diploma programs.

It is a testament to the power, influence, and wealth of the hospital associations of Pennsylvania and New Jersey that these diploma programs continue to exist. Supported by funding from the Centers for Medicare and Medicaid Services, diploma nursing education provided revenue to hospitals to ensure an intact nursing workforce, thus calming concerns about acute shortages of acute care nurses. This so-called pass-through funding for nursing education has historically been critical to maintaining diploma programs. As federal funding decreases concurrently with nursing's embrace of higher education, a perfect storm has evolved. The demands for nurses continue, even as states eliminate diploma programs.

I am under no illusion. The withdrawal of federal funding fuels closure of diploma programs. Neither concerns over the ethics of graduating young people with dead-end diplomas, nor desires to have an educated nursing workforce capable of managing the complexities of health maintenance and illness care, enter into decisions to retain or close diploma schools. The decision is always about money.

While the Temple health system did close the Episcopal Hospital Diploma School of Nursing in December 2009, it did not close its Northeastern Hospital Diploma School when that hospital was transitioned to an ambulatory practice facility in 2010. The school was retained, with administrative authority transferred to Temple University Hospital. With north Philadelphia residents at great odds with the university's closure of the hospital, the retention of the school seemed to me a token offering to the minority community to quell a potential uprising. Touted as the university's commitment to continue training local residents as nurses, the diploma school was used as a Kodak moment to bond with the host community. While I interpret this action as mere tokenism— the Community College of Philadelphia is in the area with an associate degree program in nursing—others seemed accepting of the strategy. Mindful that these diploma students cannot access the university's educational resources, including the library and Blackboard online learning, I found myself repulsed. Many of the diploma school students are racial minorities. Having been a student at Rutgers University in Newark in the late 1960s, an era of Black Power, women's rights, and protests against the war in Vietnam, I simply cannot accept disenfranchisement.

My effort to transition the remaining diploma school to a baccalaureate program continued past skirmish created by closure of the hospital. As with most change, the local community settled, adjusting over time, a testament to human resilience. My colleague responsible for our baccalaureate program and I began discussing the possibility of transitioning the diploma school to a baccalaureate program within the college shortly after it changed administrative ownership. Both the nursing director of the diploma school and the local administrator to whom she reported applauded this possibility, and thus we reinvigorated our former discussions. At one meeting, we gave each other a homework assignment. We were to investigate how the curriculum could be offered, particularly via a three-way collaboration involving my department, the faculty and administration of the diploma school, and the Community College of Philadelphia. The diploma school director and her supervisor were to explore if, and how, pass-through revenue could be retained to continue funding salaries of faculty and staff as well as nonpersonnel expenses. Pass-through funding is directed at hospital diploma schools, not degree-granting programs. Since students in the new program, as we were designing it, would continue to have clinical experiences within the Temple health system, I had urged my colleagues to simply inform the Centers for Medicare and Medicaid

Services that the curriculum would be restructured, but not the locus of field-work. If such funding could not be secured, then the possibility of this venture would evaporate.

Before we could return to discuss our homework findings, a hospital administrator met with me to discuss areas of mutual interest. When I mentioned that we were continuing our plans to transition the diploma school to a baccalaureate format, she was visibly disturbed. Indicating that the program was integral to the local community and served as a symbol of the hospital's commitment to local residents, she interrupted our planning process. The next meeting of our planning group was canceled. We were informed that a meeting of all concerned would be scheduled in the near future—she demanded compliance. Managing a large urban health system, she noted that she needed the school; it was a workforce for the hospital. As she spoke, I recalled a phrase from Lucy Drown, the superintendent of nursing at Boston City Hospital in 1899: *hospitals*, she said, *needed the bone and sinew of pupil nurses*; thus, only nursing administrators—called superintendents in that era—needed a college education. Bone and sinew—an intact workforce. In our follow-up meeting, this executive again championed the diploma school, calling the students "cognitive protoplasm," the individuals who would comprise approximately one-third of her workforce. Here were minorities at risk, their leader willing to provide them an inferior education. Self-serving and smug, she barked out orders to us, including those who did not report to her. While remaining conceptually passionate about transitioning this diploma program to a degree program, I knew I needed to let it go; it was a battle that distracted too much from our main agenda. It was a bridge too far.

When We Trust Accreditation

Pennsylvania leads the country in the number of diploma nursing schools. This distinction speaks to the power of the states's hospital association, as well as the powerlessness of its Board of Nursing. Interestingly, at a meeting in February 2011, I glimpsed the board's oppression of its own constituency: the oppressed becoming the oppressor. The context of this meeting was the *Consensus Model* for advanced practice nursing. Since the nurse practitioner certifying associations had planned on new examinations effective 2013 based on the recommendations in the consensus document, the board held the February 2011 meeting to instruct academic leaders on how to change their already board-approved programs to satisfy criteria outlined in the eligibility requirements of the new certification examinations.

I drove to the Harrisburg campus of Widener University, where the meeting was held, by myself. It was a glorious ride. Silence and time to think. My colleague did not ride with me. Perhaps tension was intruding into our relationship? The academy is such an interesting work environment, one in which supervision is abhorred and all decisions are expected to be arrived at upon the advice and counsel of all concerned—faculty and administrators alike. My colleague often disinvited me to her meetings, indicating that my presence would undermine her authority. The difference between seeking advice prior to making decisions versus seeking concurrence on decisions to be made is poorly understood by many faculties and, if understood, is frequently resented. I felt that driving separately was perhaps symbolic of her impulse to control the graduate program and, in fact, to remove my influence in it. Arriving separately, we nevertheless sat together in a stunningly beautiful circular amphitheater with several rows of comfortable chairs with arm desks. A new building, it still smelled of new carpet and exuded youthful pride. As the forty or so individuals representing graduate nurse practitioner programs settled into their seats, four Board of Nursing representatives took their places in chairs facing us, the audience. The members included a lawyer, two nursing practice advisors, and one board member who was both a certified registered nurse practitioner and a full-time faculty member. Despite the lovely, welcoming academic environment, the tone in the room became punitive as the session progressed. After a formal presentation, the board member addressed questions that had been written on index cards and given to her. Spontaneous questions were not entertained. I knew my question from the very moment I had walked into the room. Since the board requires candidates for certification as nurse practitioners to hold national certification in their specialty field, why did the board continue to demand that new academic programs preparing nurse practitioners be reviewed and approved by the board in order to be established?

Without a nanosecond of hesitation, the board member, an elderly white female with white hair swept up tightly into a bun at the back of her head, said with an authoritarian tone that there were two reasons. The first: *Because. This requirement is written in the board's regulations.* The second: Distrust. *When we trust accreditation, we may no longer require this process.* There it was, for all to hear: We do not trust ourselves, our nursing colleagues. Professional accreditation is a lengthy, self-reflective process aimed at improvement of program outcomes. I had nothing further to ask. Nor did anyone else. I did not have the courage to question this distrust of self. The authoritative tone, the wagging finger, the silence in the room reinforced my inability to engage the topic further. Clearly, my question had been addressed, and the board member put my card to the back of her index card pile, moving onto the next question. I was nonplussed, speechless. I was concerned that my question may even bring retaliation on our approved programs.

I recalled a needlepoint framed in a black border on the wall of the chief of Nursing Education at the Veterans Affairs Medical Center in East Orange, New Jersey, where I had worked after graduating from Rutgers University in 1972. A stark room with only this eight-by-ten-inch needlepoint hanging behind her desk: *Retribution Follows Sin.* Had I sinned at this meeting? Would the Temple nursing programs now be viewed differently?

Bricoleur

I talked myself into a calmer state of mind once I was in my car and back on the road to Philadelphia. Ah, cities! Cities are more forgiving, less judgmental than suburbs with their sometimes quiet unwitting despair. Inexperienced in rural life, I realized that I could not comment on the atmosphere in the many rural areas that I passed as I rode on Route 76 back to the city, a seemingly endless journey. I wondered why I bristled so vehemently when witnessing oppression imposed by some nurses on fellow nurses.

When I daydream, I sometimes toy with my necklace. When I turned sixty, my husband gave me a silver peace symbol necklace; it sparkled, a characteristic I love in jewelry. It was a peace symbol for a hippy chick on her sixtieth birthday, he said. As I played with the necklace, I recalled my college career in the late sixties—the birth of the National Organization for Women, the Black Panthers and Black Power, Students for a Democratic Society, the anti-Vietnam War protest, the general sense that change was imperative and that students could incite it. In Newark during July 1967, race riots—alternately called an insurrection movement by African Americans—tore the fabric of the city apart, exposing the despair of the black residents and the enormous disparities experienced by racial minorities, trapped in sustained poverty. It was an era of unrest, exposing inequities on multiple fronts—most prominently racial and gender. When President Richard Nixon announced the American invasion of Cambodia in April 1970, the Newark campus of Rutgers University exploded into protests. Classes were canceled, exams abandoned, with grades awarded based solely on previous work, and marches took place in the streets. Wearing the uniform of the era—hip-hugging bell-bottom jeans, T-shirts with peace symbols, and love-bead necklaces—I inhaled the spirit of the times, even as I glued myself to a library carrel, studying chemistry, anatomy and physiology, and nursing. I grew up intolerant of oppression. Any vestiges of my compliant

Catholic upbringing were snuffed out by these Rutgers college experiences, the ashes scattered by the New Jersey nursing community's attack on the nursing initiatives established by the University of Medicine and Dentistry of New Jersey during my first decade there.

I had learned to be hardy, a *bricoleur* creating *bricolage.* Hardiness and resilience are not inherent traits; they are cultivated defenses that, over time, were incorporated into my toolkit of life. I had joined UMDNJ when I was pregnant with my third child. It was a challenging pregnancy, marked by fluid retention and recurrent, crippling migraine headaches. While never diagnosed with any illness, I learned to integrate this temporary period of discomfort into my busy daily routine. I enjoyed pregnancy tremendously—an amazing, intimate, and private experience, leading to a wonderful outcome. Labeling me an elderly multigravida woman at the age of thirty-six, my physician had advised an amniocentesis to diagnose chromosomal abnormalities in the fetus, thus allowing me the option to abort if such abnormalities were identified. Since it was unlikely that I would abort, I refused the test. As I signed a document indicating that my physician had informed me of the risks associated with age and my refusal to undergo the recommended amniocentesis, I marveled at the intrusion of legal liability in health care, especially prevalent in obstetrics. I delivered my third child—a nine pound, two ounce girl—in early spring, when hardy crocuses were in bloom and the promise that March would leave like a lamb.

One week later, as my baby slept in a portable cradle on the floor in my attic office as I analyzed data to document the need for UMDNJ's planned Master of Science in Nursing program, I developed a sudden-onset headache. Experiencing a classic migraine with nausea, vomiting, extreme sensitivity to light and sound, and left-sided hemiparesis, I called my physician to ask what medication to take, since I was breastfeeding. Hours later, someone from the office called to tell me to take Tylenol. The headache escalated; I kept calling for advice. Clearly, this was the worst headache of my life. I began to slur my speech; the left-sided weakness slowly became worse. I called my physician, telling her that I was going to an emergency room, that I suspected that I was experiencing an evolving cerebral bleed—a stroke. The CT scan confirmed a cerebral bleed; the on-call neurologist at the hospital was uncertain of the cause. Ultimately, an arteriovenous malformation was diagnosed as the cause, with no surgical intervention suggested—the malformation was thought to have ruptured spontaneously. I ceased breastfeeding, stabilized neurologically, and returned home—without formal rehabilitation, given that I was considered young enough to rehab myself after receiving instructions from a physical therapist at the hospital—to my family, two young schoolchildren and my baby, who clearly preferred breast milk to Similac.

I returned to my life very quickly, but I had changed forever. Recovery from brain trauma is complex, at least partially due to the public's ignorance of brain function. Believing that a stroke impairs one's cognitive ability permanently, family members, friends, co-workers, and even some health care providers spoke to me as if I had become quite simple, unable to comprehend basic commands. My baby was taken from me—*she can't care for her baby anymore; she can't think straight*—and I retired to the couch in our living room. While still allowed to manage the family's finances, I appreciated that I was fast becoming a burden to my family. I returned full-time to UMDNJ six weeks after the birth of my daughter—Sarah Ann—while still very much in recovery. I walked with an assistive device, taking Phenobarbital for seizure control, and wearing Sears's best elastic waist sweatpants, geriatric-style Velcro high top sneakers, and T-shirts.

You're late, said President Stanley Bergen, eyeglasses teetering on the bridge of his nose, as I entered his office to review the status of our programs. We completed our agenda, and I returned to my office, locking the door and putting my head on the desk for a few minutes, before I delved into the next steps to be taken to start programs at the university.

My stroke was an inconvenience, but I had an aggressive agenda. Knowing that the brain's elasticity could accommodate growth, I became confident that I could achieve my goals at UMDNJ—to start academic nursing programs and to establish a separate School of Nursing. There was only going forward. I would never be late again.

At my back was my intellectual liberation at New York University, where I learned there simply was no thought you couldn't think. Ahead was the nursing community's solid block of opposition to UMDNJ's venture into academic nursing. And there was my stroke, a private physical phenomenon that I worked to manage, and eventually to control the consequences, including seizures. My 1987 stroke was known within the nursing community. Nurse leaders' anger at Stanley Bergen's perceived intrusion into nursing education, coupled with knowledge of my health status, fueled hate speech. At a national nursing conference, I was coined Bergen's *"brain-dead whore."* While I occasionally toyed with the idea of suing these individuals for defamation of character, I never did. Freed to be me, I gradually became acquainted more fully with my own values and strengths. I planned to recover fully, and quickly. I read Steve Fishman's 1990 story, *Bomb in the Brain*, and knew that others had had this experience, and continued to live and contribute. Hippie chick from the sixties, my priorities shifted radically. My bar for tolerating oppression was reset on low, a characteristic that will remain with me for the rest of my life. I became very hardy.

When my colleague and I reviewed the Pennsylvania Board of Nursing's materials from the special meeting held in February 2011, we understood what we needed to do for compliance. The board member's mistrust of nursing's accreditation processes would not change in the near future. I seemed to be the sole complainant. My colleague urged, *just do what they want, it's easier that way.* Yes, it is easier to accept oppression than to fight it; compliance trumps the ambiguity of risk, the loneliness of challenge. My colleague promised to fill out the board's forms diligently.

One can self-liberate from oppression. Liberation takes practice. The School of Nursing at UMDNJ was established in 1997, and programs became accredited by the National League for Nursing Accreditation Commission (NLNAC). Since accreditors are us—that is, nurses—I had assumed a very collegial approach to the process of accreditation. Surely, if we conformed to the spirit of accreditation, then any deviance from standards could be logically described and accepted by accreditors. The nursing programs were reevaluated for continued accreditation in 2002. In my last year as dean of the school, I worked with faculty on our self-study, and literally drove it—all multiple copies, each one-and-a-half-inches thick—to the NLNAC headquarters in New York. But this self-study included an indiscretion on my part. I had recruited and employed several registered nurses for faculty positions who held graduate degrees in diverse fields, including one with a Master of Public Health and others with non-nursing doctoral degrees. Since the NLNAC requires that faculty require a minimum of a master's degree in nursing, my recruitment of nurses with other degrees was categorized as noncompliant.

My experiences at UMDNJ had taught me the value of intellectual diversity. I learned more about my own field when I needed to articulate it to others at deans' meetings at UMDNJ. What would nursing offer to a multidisciplinary care team in the prison system, for example? I found my voice and my discipline's unique contributions to health care delivery through conversations with physicians, dentists, public health professionals, and biomedical scientists. Taking it one step further, I began to appreciate a diverse nursing faculty. Nurses with doctorates in nursing, or public health, or public administration, or education, or other fields. Or, non-nurses with doctorates in fields such as statistics or psychometrics. Different viewpoints yield different perspectives on one topic; a richness of thought is brought to any topic through a diversely educated faculty. It is quite difficult to maintain nursing's grip on an incestuous educational standard in the face of a rich pool of intellectual talent. As I drove through the Holland Tunnel to the NLNAC on Broadway in New York City on a warm, sunny day in June 2002, I felt accomplished and proud. As I exited as dean, the programs were safely on their way to reaccreditation, with a solid, diverse faculty and excellent outcomes. On my return after a short vacation, my former secretary told me that the interim dean who replaced me was concerned about the inclusion of faculty with non-nursing master's degrees being included in the self-study; therefore, she had the documents returned to UMDNJ. The names and curriculum vitae of the offending faculty were removed, and the amended self-study was forwarded to the agency. In short order, the offending faculty members were thus not reappointed. The pull toward compliance is incredibly strong; the resultant intellectual narrowness flourishes. Nursing's modernist orientation, a teleological view opposing context, is frequently cruel.

While researching the history of nursing in New Jersey, I was fortunate to come across the interesting aberrancy of a training school for nursing in Waltham, Massachusetts, at the turn of the twentieth century. The Waltham school rotated its pupil nurses between hospital units and homes to get diverse clinical experiences, as noted in Alfred Worcester's papers located in the archives of Harvard University's Library of Medicine. In the late nineteenth century, states initiated registration of nurses on the basis of years of service in hospital-based training programs, with specific rotations in clinical areas. State registration was connected to hospital education, with home care the exclusive domain of graduate nurses. Pupils trained exclusively in hospitals as a workforce; graduates were employed exclusively in private duty home nursing. Education absent of home context, the modern factory of health—the hospital— was assured a sustained workforce reified through state registration. While the Waltham school was praised by local nurse leaders at that time, the school did ultimately close since its graduates were not deemed eligible for registered nurse licensure. At a hearing reported in *The Trained Nurse and Hospital Review* (January 1914) on the subject of the school's perceived defiance regarding curriculum design for licensure eligibility, the nurse leader of the National Organization of Public Health Nursing indicated that nursing must hold firm to registration standards, questioning, *Would you have us change our standards which control all the country?* The Waltham administrators responded *yes,* as I would today. The Waltham training school had also served as the focal point for a possible school of nursing at Harvard University. When Harvard University's young president, Charles Elliot, considered establishing a school of nursing in the early twentieth century patterned after the Waltham school, nurse leaders at the time objected. The hospital was idolatrized; as America underwent

Harvardization, nursing education remained secluded in hospitals, under close management first by medicine and hospital administrators, and then by nurse leaders. As Michel Foucault hypothesized in *Discipline and Punish: The Birth of the Prison* (1977), the oppressed become oppressors—in the twenty-first century, as in the twentieth century. The teleological fix was in.

An Attorney for Nursing

On January 15, 1992, the nurse practitioner/clinical nurse specialist bill. became law in New Jersey, signed by Governor James Florio (Chapter 377, *Laws of New Jersey,* 1991). *Fran,* said Julie, *we have to design a collaborative practice agreement for prescriptive authority.* Julie was a young attorney I had recruited to manage the UMDNJ School of Nursing's myriad clinical affiliation agreements and academic partnerships. Julia—smart, tall, angular, and with a razor sharp, biting edge both in tone and language—was right. With each win, more work was required. And each win demanded increasing vigilance, recognizing that not all physicians, or for that matter not all nurses, endorsed the legislation. Julie crafted two agreements—one for internal physicians and a second for physicians external to the university. As a woman lawyer, Julie understood paternalism, power, and control. At one Board of Nursing meeting, Julie was assumed to be a secretary, simply because she took notes. Her prickly hypervigilance sometimes got in her way, distracting her, resulting in long conversations about gender and power. Despite this, her written documents were stellar, receiving compliments from the UMDNJ legal team. When I first recruited a lawyer for the school, a minor flurry of discontent evolved between me and the legal team. Why did I think it necessary to have a lawyer internal to the school? Didn't the university's legal department adequately address any nursing legal issues? Eventually, the tension dissipated. I needed legal advice just as routinely as I needed our finance staff to manage our budget. I needed to be very, very alert to medicine's potential landmines to sabotage nursing's growing independence. My practice in the fast track in the Emergency Department of University Hospital was signed by physicians in this clinical area, not with a department at New Jersey Medical School. Only the osteopathic school on the Stratford campus was receptive. (That dean's sister was a nurse practitioner.) Monitoring assembly and senate bills, remaining in routine communication with the political action arm of the New Jersey State Nurses Association, and monitoring regulations promulgated by the Board of Nursing was a full-time position in itself. Nursing's vigilance was warranted in an environment frequently hostile to a post-modern view of health care delivery.

Julie's collaborative practice agreements (CPA) were simple and conformed to requirements spelled out in regulations concerning joint protocols. While at UMDNJ, I had a fully executed CPA with an osteopathic physician in Stratford. Dark hair, beautifully tailored suits, highly polished Italian shoes; the osteopath was a charming and confident collaborator, colleague, and friend. The CPA outlined my prescriptive practice with the osteopath as the collaborating physician; it also included general provisions regarding regulated mandates such as annual review of the CPA, standards for clinical practice, records maintenance, consultation and referral requirements, and emergency care protocols. He signed the CPA without careful scrutiny—eager to work with me in the Camden Community Health Center. While at the center, I occasionally referred patients to him, including a few who were uninsured. He triaged referred patients, as needed, to specialists within the school. He never refused a patient; in fact, his department would help to supply the center with sample medications as needed. My relationship with my osteopathic colleague also included interdisciplinary education of osteopathic students and nurse practitioner students. It is interesting that relationships such as those exemplified in CPAs are so very dependent on the personalities and characteristics of the individuals involved. Within the university, UMDNJ leaders could not orchestrate institutional policy regarding CPAs; such agreements could only be driven at the individual level. As the president said casually at a celebratory event, *I like to watch the schools battle over matters involving primary care delivery.* One allopathic dean assured me that he reigned, not ruled. Therefore, I would have to fend for myself to convince individual physicians to sign CPAs. I have subsequently wondered if older, more mature organizations might be capable of instituting policy to facilitate matters such as interdisciplinary education, or collaborative practice for primary care. Perhaps not, since at the end of the day, execution of policy is dependent on the people in place, complete with their biases and greed.

At UMDNJ in the 1990s, Julie was successful in crafting template CPAs for nurse practitioner faculty. At Temple University in 2008, Nancy Rothman deftly managed CPAs for me with two physicians involved with the network of nurse-managed health centers in Philadelphia. The Pennsylvania Board of Nursing requires that a collaborative agreement between a nurse practitioner and a supervising physician be filed with the board in order for a CRNP Prescriptive Authority license to be issued by the board. One can be certified as a registered nurse practitioner in Pennsylvania, but to practice prescriptive authority, the board must also issue a prescriptive authority license. To practice primary care with prescriptive practice in Pennsylvania, I needed to be a licensed CRNP in adult health and to hold a separate CRNP Prescriptive Authority license naming specifically my collaborating physician. Additionally, as is the case with anyone prescribing controlled dangerous substances, I needed to obtain a Drug Enforcement Administration (DEA) number through the U.S. Department of Justice. In turn, the collaborating physician must comply with corollary regulations promulgated by the Board of Medical Examiners. This board mandates that at any time a physician may not supervise more than four CRNPs who prescribe and dispense drugs (Pennsylvania State Board of Medical Examiners, §18.57). Prescribing medications is equated with primary care.

School-Based Health: An Example of Collaborative Practice

In March 2011, I hosted a meeting at Temple University of several individuals very interested in encouraging my department to expand our reach into the Philadelphia school system. In September 2010, through the relationships cultivated by Nancy Rothman, our department assumed the function of school nurse at the Pan American Academy School in North Philadelphia. At that time, this charter school had incrementally increased classes from kindergarten to sixth grade, with a student census of over four hundred. Since charter schools must conform to Department of Education regulations, this school required an on-site school nurse to implement functions required by the department. The nursing department had accepted a contract from the National Nursing Centers Consortium (NNCC), supported also by the Public Health Management Corporation (PHMC). We received funding to hire a full-time nurse practitioner, with the goal of transitioning the school nurse office into a primary care center to service the children, their families, and the general neighborhood. Such a plan was congruent with the health care reform legislation—that is, to provide accessible primary care delivery within schools, hypothesizing that absentee rates would decline and academic success indices would rise. Here was a wonderful idea, if only on a shoestring budget. But Nancy and I undertook it anyway.

In summer 2010, when the grant was funded, Nancy and I began one of the most arduous recruitment efforts we have ever undertaken. How difficult would it be to attract a pediatric or family nurse practitioner to work in a North Philadelphia school system, blending the roles of school nurse and primary care provider in an effort to provide local, accessible care? It turned out to be very difficult. Interview after interview, our offer of the position was rejected. There were enough candidates; it was more a combination of salary and neighborhood that ultimately was unattractive. As it crept closer and closer to the end of August, Nancy and I lost sleep. Nancy then remembered her roommate from nursing school—a retired school nurse with decades of experience in the Philadelphia school system.

Nancy charmed her friend to join us as a consultant. Within a few days of the first phone call, Nancy's friend was on duty at the Pan American Academy, in the narrow, long, rectangular room referred to as the Wellness Center. The school itself occupied an old, magnificent four-story building, with large rooms and walls thick with paint applied over many years. The walls were now all colorful, light blues, yellow, pink, and other eye-catching colors. The Academy operated through a partnership with Congreso de Latinos Unidos, a community-based nonprofit organization that contributed social services on site. A major goal of the Academy and Congreso was to transition the school nurse program to a primary care site, with Congreso's own health center—a federally qualified health center—partnering to provide continuous health services beyond school hours. Our mission was therefore twofold: to provide essential school nurse functions; and to expand services to primary care delivery via pediatric or family nurse practitioner services. With her colleague on board, Nancy quickly galvanized her rich network of colleagues and we began to think of other options. By the end of the first month of the school year, we had three nurse practitioners in place, each part time, under the guidance of our part-time consultant. Job sharing this position, the three nurse practitioners now needed a collaborative practice agreement with a pediatrician in order to provide primary care on site. They also needed to receive emergency certification as school nurses through the Department of Education, with the full appreciation that they would ultimately have to complete a school nurse certification program.

We went to our colleagues within the Temple University School of Medicine to form a collaborative practice agreement with the Department of Pediatrics. It seemed reasonable to Nancy and me that we should first approach our family, rather than go to Thomas Jefferson Hospital where several of our other collaborating physicians were affiliated. The department chair of pediatrics was very agreeable to signing a collaborative practice agreement, as was one of his faculty members, a young female pediatrician eager for involvement in the school system. Internal politics, drama over payment for the collaborating physician, and simple inertia impeded progress for months. September, October, November, December, January, February—six months' delay, at one point over who should sign the agreement. Once signed, the agreement was then forwarded to the Pennsylvania State Board of Nursing so that the nurse practitioners at the Academy would receive the CRNP prescriptive authority licenses, which included the pediatrician's name. As the spring semester of our first school year came to a close, these licenses had not yet been returned to the CRNPs. The delays in getting these licenses back during year one at the Academy, therefore, resulted in a domino effect. Without the licenses in hand, PHMC could not go to health insurance providers—Keystone Mercy and Health Partners—and seek a rate for CRNP primary care services provided at the Academy. The CRNPs managed ill children or triaged them to outside providers. Once a rate is established, and assuming that the CRNPs are also appropriately credentialed by the health insurance companies as primary care providers, PHMC could bill these insurers for the services provided. Billing: the final frontier. To get to the stage of being able to bill is to get to the finish line. Crossing the line means that revenue from clinical services billed has been received. The power plays associated with academic politics delayed full execution of the collaborative agreement; this, in turn, delayed receipt of Board of Nursing–approved CRNP prescriptive authority licenses, which delayed negotiation of insurance rates and, thus, no billing or receiving of clinical income could take place for at least a year. What could have taken a few days took academic semesters.

As I sat in our conference room, a smart classroom outfitted with tables and chairs that fit together like Lincoln logs, and thus always seemed untidy and in disarray, our first year at the Pan American Academy flashed through my consciousness. I had taken our faculty there for an on-site faculty meeting, my intent to rally enthusiasm for the initiative. They did not require rallying; they were already on board—nurses doing community work consistent with Temple's urban mission. (An amazing cohort of nursing faculty.) We had a department comprised of almost all non-tenure track faculty, so very vulnerable in a larger university system enamored only with tenure-track, or tenured, faculty. And, like most nurses, they were quite unfamiliar with the no margin, no mission cornerstone of care delivery. An administrator from the National Nursing Centers Consortium, a representative from a large nonprofit health institute, and a board member of a Philadelphia foundation concerned with school-based health care joined Nancy and me at our conference table. Forever gracious and extremely adept at navigating tricky terrain, Nancy urged everyone to enjoy an early lunch, since our meeting might interrupt their lunch times. The representative from the foundation, a petite brunette with a sculpted pageboy hairdo, placed her iPhone and iPad on the table before her, intermittently checking sites and e-mail prior to the start of our meeting. In paced sentences and very articulate speech, she smiled warmly, detailing with passion the need for school nurse help at two other private schools recently established in Philadelphia, in close geographic proximity to the Pan American Academy. These two new schools, together with an approximate enrollment for fall 2011 of two hundred students, did not yet enjoy on site health services. The Nursing Center Consortium administrator, wearing her sharp, vigilant businesswoman hat, noted that these schools did not have to comply with Board of Education regulations since they were private. *Not that we wouldn't give quality service*, she was quick to state. The foundation representative requested that we consider replicating our work at these two new schools, hiring one family or pediatric nurse practitioner who would again be under the tutelage of Barbara, who would be now able to leave the Pan American Academy to assist a new nurse practitioner brought on board to implement the new initiative. One person present indicated that funds would be available to support the new initiative, even though we were experiencing a funding deficit for the Pan American effort in its first year of operation.

I felt a vague unease as our meeting progressed. As the Nursing Centers Consortium administrator leaned forward in her chair, she asked if our nurse practitioner students could provide services at the new schools: *Why are we supporting these programs if the students can't help?* she asked, with a furrowed brow. Her question was core to understanding the differences between graduate nurse practitioner students and graduate medical students. Graduate medical students, serving as residents in acute care hospitals, provide direct care under the supervision of an attending physician. Graduate nurse practitioner students, the majority full-time employees attending evening courses on a part-time basis, were shifting roles from nursing to primary care—diagnosing and managing disease, as well as providing health promotion services. Our students, I said, were at Temple to learn, not to provide service without an accompanying educational benefit. At neither the undergraduate nor graduate level did our students serve as care providers. I could not obligate our students to service at any school, irrespective of the evidence that such initiatives lent to the validity and credibility of the school-based, nurse-managed health center effort. While our students could supplement service through their student role, they could not be counted on as the workforce on any regular basis. As we continued to discuss options, we expressed impatience with the Board of Nursing's sluggish bureaucracy, its general negativity, and our sense that it erected barriers to nurse practitioner practice when none need exist. A self-imposed restriction on trade. Waving her hand, she noted that it was *so much easier to work with physicians!*

I had been in such a dilemma before. In 1996, Stanley Bergen, the president of the University of Medicine and Dentistry of New Jersey, had invited me to provide health services at the Saint Columba Neighborhood Club, a community-based Hispanic organization located on Pennsylvania Avenue in Newark. *This is your opportunity,* he had said, to do what I had been advocating—an opportunity for nurse practitioners to provide direct primary care. None of the university's three medical schools were interested in working at Saint Columba's, housed in a desperately impoverished area of the city, with a large indigent, uninsured, or underinsured population. I agreed to work with the organization, placing two full-time professional staff in two rooms designated as the health center. We obtained funding from the Robert Wood Johnson Foundation to support our initiatives, and the Hispanic chief executive officer of our University Hospital provided us with the recurring clinical supplies needed on a monthly basis. Students rotated through the center, and health education programs were offered at the Catholic grammar school associated with Saint Columba's. It was a wonderful success; it was also an abysmal failure.

As an academic fieldwork program, the Saint Columba Neighborhood Club health center sponsored by the school of nursing provided students and faculty alike with teaching-learning programs in community health that were practical and outcomes oriented. We generated data for multiple evidence-based research projects. From a service delivery perspective, I see now, with the clarity of hindsight, that we were amazingly immature regarding health care reimbursement. Julie, my staff lawyer, obtained a card-swiping machine by which to identify patients' health insurance information. We did not know even the basics of reimbursement. While we did have a Board of Trustees–approved Nursing Faculty Practice Plan, we were ignorant of the detailed mechanics involved in having nurse practitioners credentialed by health insurance companies who had Medicaid plans. We never visited health insurance companies to negotiate a rate of payment for nurse practitioners providing services at the Saint Columba center. We did not know of the International Statistical Classification of Diseases and Related Health Problems list of codes for billing purposes; nor were we familiar with the American Medical Association's Current Procedural Terminology (CPT) codes for billing patient encounters. If we had understood the mechanics of coding and billing, then another practical matter might have surfaced: Would it have been financially lucrative enough for the university to support the infrastructure necessary at the center to bill for the services provided by nurse practitioners? Again, I have sometimes looked back at my Saint Columba days with both pride and embarrassment: pride at our outcomes in that blighted neighborhood; embarrassment at my naiveté.

Of course, the president could count on me to accept his invitation— nursing could always be pointed to for examples of the university's involvement in our host community: hard work, extensive relationship building, and hours spent in sophisticated volunteerism, often at the cost of time spent in research or other scholarly pursuits. At Saint Columba we provided primary health care, but not primary care; and, we referred patients to the medical school for needed primary care or specialty care—the money following the physician, billing for health promotion and disease prevention services not yet possible.

My Saint Columba experience occurred at the same general time when Medicaid became managed, with Medicaid patients able to choose primary care providers. Physicians scrambled to enroll Medicaid patients in their practices, stealing away the young pregnant women previously managed exclusively by the nurse midwifery program at the university. These patients, to the stunned amazement of the midwifery faculty, left in droves to be cared for by the very physicians who previously closed their doors to them. In fact, the move to steal this patient population was so vicious that the medical school implemented a policy that prevented the midwives from caring for these patients within a certain radius of the university. The midwives were shut down, their patients moving to the Doctor's Office Complex on the campus—a new building— complete with the prestige and white lab coats of physicians. Accustomed to medicine's greed, the midwives regrouped. They moved their practice to another health system outside of the university. A major hiccup, the university's medical school's actions gave the midwives an opportunity to move to the private sector—a health system committed to quality care and to financial success. In the end, the midwives managed well. Both their educational program— which was totally dependent on their practice plan—and their clinical services survived, and thrived. The midwives, however, had been disenfranchised from the university; an environment had been created that placed midwifery faculty on the fringe, cruelly discarded. The medical school was allowed to behave in this manner, a fact illustrating the institution's inability—or unwillingness—to restrain physicians' greed and to curb arrogance.

Now, years later, at Temple University, I faced this phenomenon again, but in the academic, not the clinical, arena. In 2006, the nursing and medical faculty jointly provided a simulation learning center; that is, a practice laboratory with computerized manikin patients pre-programmed to illustrate a variety of common acute illnesses. The center, in fact, was first initiated by a nursing faculty member who obtained grant funding to purchase a Simulation "Man"—an investment of close to $40,000. A great success—as measured by faculty and student satisfaction—and an example of interdisciplinary education, the center expanded and was eventually moved in 2009 to a larger site in a newly constructed medical school building. Nursing's equipment moved to the new site. One faculty administrator, an intellectually gifted, quiet, and highly skilled person, applauded the move. She rolled up her sleeves and transported equipment on gurneys, carefully moving manikins and associated supplies across

Broad Street, a wide, heavily trafficked road bordered on one corner by the hospital and the medical and health professions' schools on the others. The original designer of the center constructed patient simulation scenarios appropriate to both medical and nursing students. She was truly thrilled with the center's new location. Once there, the tsunami wave of greed hit, and hit again. Nursing would now be charged an hourly fee to use the Simulation Center. We would need to submit our requests to use the center well in advance, with nursing's requests considered only after medicine's requests were considered. We would have to pay to use our equipment, our scenarios, perhaps at inconvenient times. And, to use the standardized patient section of the center for our graduate students, the cost to my department for a three-day program was close to $6,000.

My rage was uncontrollable and I was alone in this. The fee was paid. When I sought a new fee to be charged to students to pay for these costs in future years, the members of the university fee committee didn't blink. *Well,* said one member of the committee, *the medical school's costs have to be met.* The fee charged by the medical school was addressed quickly, without discussion or challenge. Two weeks later I informed the medical school that I was taking nursing's Sim Man back home, to our Nursing Resource Center. My rage quieted with this action. I would ask Sandy to ride our equipment back across Broad Street, home to our students, no fees, no charge-backs, and no inequities. From 1996 to 2011, from midwives' practice to nurse practitioner education, there has been little change in medicine's hierarchical orientation or quest for resources. My rage is uncontrollable.

Can the Answer Be No?

Against the backdrop of my Saint Columba experiences and my years of adventures with medicine, the Temple proposal in 2011 to extend school-based health services to two Philadelphia private schools was easier to manage. Without secure funding, the program could not be established. At the Academy charter school, billing for primary care services offered by nurse practitioners dually certified as school nurses could eventually be undertaken once prescriptive authority licenses were obtained and health insurance rates were negotiated with companies offering Medicaid contracts. Students would not be counted on for service, only for supplemental assistance. Why couldn't I simply say *no* at the very beginning of the conversation, if funding was not secure? Thirty-nine years into nursing—and by now quite familiar with nursing's history—I believe I have some rudimentary understanding of nursing's inability to say no. Nurses' goals have traditionally been to achieve the goals of others, be they physicians, hospital administrators, or patients and their families. Monastic in origin, nursing's roots are embedded in compliance, subservience, and dependent functioning. Nurses have historically fought collective bargaining as a tool of the uneducated, technical worker, not to be confused with professional behaviors and self-regulation. Trained in hospitals as an institutional workforce, nurses gained a toehold in higher education only in the mid-twentieth century, long after the Harvardization of America had taken place. Without money, there is no chance for mission; only missionary work and volunteerism remain, neither one capable of fast-forwarding nurse practitioners as credentialed primary care providers on insurance panels. Nurses are easy prey to target for volunteer work in poor urban environments.

Our meeting ended on an affable note. Nancy and I would explore possible planned student fieldwork experiences at these school sites, and the National Nursing Centers Consortium would renew its efforts to secure funding. While our academic mission often intertwined with service initiatives, it was clear that students couldn't be sacrificed to meet patients' needs. Education had to matter in nursing, particularly if we intended to bill for registered nurse as well as nurse practitioner services. I share the National Nursing Centers Consortium administrator's impatience with Board of Nursing mandates. Despite my appreciation of her efforts to advance the nurse practitioner movement, however, I knew that I needed to balance these initiatives with the protection of our students involved in nurse practitioner education. In residency, graduate medical students are paid; graduate nursing students are not.

Saying no is complex and uncomfortable. As I had to learn hardiness, I also had to learn to say no. *Why can't this program come under the name of New Jersey Medical School,* queried the senior vice president for academic affairs at UMDNJ in 1998. Adding that I could still run the program, but it should be offered by the medical school instead of the nursing school, this official, sitting tall and pompous, his ingratiating language attempted to persuade me to come to my senses, to recognize that this proposed program needed to emanate from a more prestigious unit within the university. I could still run the program, he offered, but just let the UMDNJ degree partner to this interinstitutional venture be the medical school. Remain invisible and busy, doing the work, but without public recognition. Just be a girl, dammit! Our conversation was tense, and the stakes were high for me and my fledgling school of nursing, a unit very alive with ideas, and very close to the street level of health care delivery. *No,* I said, *the answer is no.* I sat at the small conference table, my hands gripping my chair, my mind racing. What else should I say? I ended our meeting abruptly; there was nothing left to say. For several years, I had spearheaded the establishment of a new PhD program in Urban Systems. The program had been designed as an interinstitutional, multidisciplinary initiative involving Rutgers University and the New Jersey Institute of Technology. The goal of the program was to offer three tracks—one in urban health, one in urban education, and one in urban environment. My life and work in New Jersey cities— Newark and Camden—framed my understanding that the interaction of city systems was the complex phenomenon at the heart of the poor health indices of urban minorities. Irrespective of the central presence of academic health centers in cities, health indices of minorities have remained consistently poor for decades, as noted in *Healthy People 2010*, and *2020*. Poverty, deeply embedded in the lives, thinking, and culture of city residents, is evidenced daily in urban university hospitals. Even as Newark policemen direct university employees safely out of parking lots at 5 P.M. every evening at UMDNJ, residents remain in a city marked by violence, disease, and depression. No way out, no policeman to help them exit. Newark needed more.

In 1998, the PhD program was approved by the UMDNJ Board of Trustees, with the School of Nursing named as the unit responsible for the track in urban health. In 2010, I received a thank you card for a nurse who had just received her PhD in Urban Systems, with a specialization in urban health; she had been aware of the program's difficult gestation period, and simply thanked me for staying with it. Adamant that she did not want a PhD in nursing—she thought such programs would give her more of the same—she had chosen our program for its multidisciplinary nature. As I read her card, more than a decade after the battles had been won, I felt again the intense anger and pain of that time, recalling that I had been called *just a clinician* and incapable of offering such a highly complex program. The bias against nursing is palpable, with the paternalism of medicine continuing to exist into the twenty-first century, made more complex by nursing's sustained inability to clarify its scope of practice based on education. To cull out an independent role in health care delivery, nursing must finally say no to invisibility.

Urban Systems

Joe, a forty-eight-year-old male homeless resident living in a large shelter in Philadelphia, was one of my first patients at the Mary Howard Health Center. Big, with the muscular build of a life-long weightlifter, Joe was an angry man who alternated living in shelters with prison stays. Low back pain was his presenting complaint, with anger management the most pressing need; he also had a complex history of drug and alcohol use and hypertension. When had his back pain started? Joe hesitated, then responded by telling me about his maltreatment during one prison stay, which had resulted in trauma to his back. His straight-leg raise test was positive, indicating a possible underlying herniated disk. Joe was sent for X-rays and subsequently for neurologic evaluation; his magnetic resonance imaging (MRI) test revealed radiculopathy in the lower lumbar region. He received physical therapy and pain management; his low back pain decreased but his anger remained. Our psychiatric mental health nurse practitioner evaluated him, and placed him on medication.

Approximately one year later, Joe's primary care visits have changed in character. Joe had become quite integrated into the shelter where he resided, often helping at the front desk, performing triage duties, helping to control unruly residents, participating in group sessions. He reunited with a former girlfriend, asking me for Viagra. His multiple medications for hypertension management had left him, as he said, *in real trouble!* Unable to receive Viagra or any other medication for erectile dysfunction due to restrictions imposed by his health insurance, Joe and I found alternate solutions—candles, good food, music, a romantic environment. Fortunately, he came back reporting that romance worked! Joe was offered a job at the shelter, to serve as their front desk area helper—their guard to manage crowd control and other general duties. *If I do this, then I'd be off of welfare.* He was worried; this job offer was terribly confusing. Should he work? He had never had a job. No one in his family had had jobs; he recalls his family was always on welfare and had Medicaid benefits. He was afraid; he wanted my opinion. I told him only that I loved work; that I loved earning money and having my own income; that income was liberating. *Maybe I should take this job,* Joe pondered. *You can break this cycle,* I told him. Rather than spending a few more years on trying to win a case for receipt of Social Security Disability income, supported by court-appointed young lawyers, try employment. A new and frightening world for Joe, but he left the office indicating that he would take the shelter job, and then find an apartment for himself and his girlfriend.

Urban systems. I am glad that I learned to say no to power.

Chapter 5

Context, Data, and Judgment

When Is Enough, Enough?

While illness can be managed by treatment algorithms, managing health is quite the contrary. People are complex. Often, their medical problem is presented as simply an admission ticket to the system, where they subtly hope for more. Co-managing pain in a homeless, hypertensive patient injured in a fall requires the single commodity impossible to provide in our health care system: time. My experiences in Philadelphia's Mary Howard Health Center grounded me in the stark lexicon of reimbursement. Billing encounters—complete with boxes to check for level of patient complexity, diagnostic coding, interventions taken, and counseling provided—drive center funding. In addition, types of encounters—routine physical examinations, illness visits, and others—link to preestablished time units. *Fifteen minutes for a follow-up visit? Twenty minutes for a physical examination?* Insurers hope for high productivity standards, perhaps four patient encounters per hour, twenty-four in a six-hour clinical day. As time per visit decreases, use of expensive diagnostic testing increases. Listening to patients' health narratives and conducting physical examinations shred appoint schedules. Fears of malpractice haunt these visits. Within the capitalistic framework of efficiency, caring in context is burdensome. As health insurance reforms are undertaken, health care may change, with accountable care organizations focusing on patient-centeredness. Such a shift, however, may ultimately be limited in quality outcomes if the imperious intellectus orientation of medicine remains with the physician as the lead provider. The dualisms of hierarchy need to be shattered, disrupting the ownership of health care by insurers and

leveling the primary care provider field. At Mary Howard, Cynthia, a sixty-year-old depressed patient with multiple comorbidities, leads her care. *It is my life, isn't it?* she asks. Yes, it is her life, but managing her health with her as lead took time, courage, and risk. How would a jury of my peers evaluate my care? Who, exactly, are my peers?

*

In early spring of 2001, on a beautiful day, an unusual tableau of individuals sat together in the New York City office of Ambassador Joseph Mutaboba, permanent representative of Rwanda to the United Nations. As members of a health mission team going to Rwanda in May 2001, my colleague Carolyn and I had questions about licensure and regulation of nursing practice in that country. Would we be allowed to provide primary care in Rwanda? Should we carry with us any documentation authorizing us to provide health care in Rwanda, given that we had not been educated or licensed in that country? Were there any regulatory barriers to our practicing in Rwanda? Nurse practitioners had just won a prolonged battle in New Jersey in the late twentieth century to practice primary care with prescriptive authority. As we prepared for our trip to Rwanda, we felt compelled to ask these questions, our minds vigilant and accustomed to looking around corners for opposition to our practice. Additionally, Rwanda was fragile politically, with a new government; would we be at risk as foreigners practicing primary care or episodic care if we did not carry with us proper documentation authorizing us to do so? It was a beautiful day, and we were afraid.

Global Health—An Opportunity

The office was sparsely furnished, with a large wooden desk filling most of the room. A photograph of Rwanda's president—Paul Kagame—hung crookedly in a cheap frame on the wall behind the desk. With a musty aroma filling the room, visitors get the sense that this office is used infrequently. My mental picture of ambassadorships—a very romantic one framed by Hollywood movies—shattered. The tall, thin, impeccably groomed man sitting at his desk exuded a calm, patient, and gentle aura as he folded his hands and leaned forward to talk with us, listening intensely to the goals of our mission and our concerns about regulations. Prior to his present appointment, Mr. Mutaboba, with his master of philosophy degree in library and information science from North London University, had played an active role in his country's security-sector reform process. With a beautiful command of English, and a very slight, almost imperceptible British accent, he told us that no, he did not see any reason for us to be concerned; there were no barriers to our giving health care in Rwanda. Our licenses to practice here in the United States would be adequate documentation for us to care for his people in Rwanda. He spoke softly, and very slowly. *Do what you are capable of doing*, he urged us, *my people need care*. As he spoke, the office seemed to get darker, even gloomy; the incredible sadness in his voice laying bare, perhaps for the first time for me, the human consequences attendant to Rwanda's hundred-day genocide in 1994.

It was a flashpoint moment. My sense of shame and embarrassment about my self-protective urgency to be held harmless from the potential risk of practicing in Rwanda with only my New Jersey license was compounded by an equally strong pull to help, irrespective of professional risk. I felt small in his presence. Racing, conflicting conversations occurred quickly in my head. Surely Newark and Camden needed as much, if not more, health services help than Rwanda. As our conversation closed, he gave each of us copies of a child's story about the mountain gorillas of Rwanda; in the preface, Ambassador Mutaboba had written that in the twentieth century, the world had witnessed the worst wars and genocides, including the one in Rwanda in 1994, "but the children at the beginning of this millennium may be our best hope for peace and lasting prosperity." Mutaboba's reference to Rwanda's genocide in Marc D. Gutekunst's 2000 book *Maji and the Mountain Gorillas of Rwanda* was tangential; veiled language embedded in his inscription in my copy of this children's book: *With my prayers and thanks, Joseph Mutaboba*. I struggled with this experience for weeks prior to going to Rwanda. Even though I had spent my life in the toughest parts of tough cities, I couldn't fathom the hate that had been unleashed in Rwanda.

I grew up in a Scottish household, with parents born in Dumbarton, Scotland, in the early twentieth century. Young children during World War I, they had felt the full impact of World War II—the Big One, as they called to it. My mother served as an army driver, tooling around Europe and Great Britain, carrying generals to and from battle sites. As a frail elderly Alzheimer's resident in a nursing home in Berkeley Heights, New Jersey, in the late 1990s, she relived the war daily, directing nursing staff to watch the marching front line from her window, to be on duty and vigilant. As a first-generation American with British parents, I had heard of "darkies"—a term used to describe Indians and Pakistanis—and my father's trips to Burma and other countries that seemed exotic. My mother exuded the pride of the British Empire, defensive of its history of colonization; my father, on the other hand, was a quiet rebel against the empire, teasing my mother that she should go back if it was so good there.

While Britain did not colonize Rwanda, its imperial presence was clearly experienced on the African continent from the Cape to Cairo, with trade interests and Christianizing the natives paramount.

I was deeply unsettled by the internal tension I experienced over why I had agreed to the mission trip to Rwanda. At the time, I was dean of the School of Nursing at the University of Medicine and Dentistry of New Jersey (UMDNJ), and Carolyn was the assistant dean for our Stratford campus. The trip was not a university-sponsored effort; rather, it was part of the social mission of Carolyn's church to give back to society on a global scale. Ten years later, I appreciate that I went on this trip out of loyalty to Carolyn, and also because of embarrassment about my British heritage of centuries of cruel colonization of Africa. "Darkies" were not equal to humans, at least not to the British and, maybe, not to many Americans, either. This trip met my personal need to visit Africa, to see Africans in their own country and to appreciate what it might feel like to be a minority.

Carolyn did not go to Rwanda. She had sustained a complex series of leg fractures during a skiing accident and was not fully weight-bearing by the time of the trip. A second UMDNJ colleague, who had also been a part of the original team, did not go either, due to pressures from her family about the political risks in Rwanda. The team included a physician assistant, a minister, a psychologist, a traveling physician, a retired engineer, and several others, including a student. The physician assistant, Rosa, worked in the emergency room of UMDNJ's University Hospital in Newark; we had worked together for some time, a fact that served us well as we set up temporary clinics in several Rwandan villages.

I had never faced such an unknown. During our flights to Europe and then to Kigali Airport in Rwanda, I voraciously read my book of infectious disease management. Unfamiliar with the diagnosis and management of malaria, yellow fever, bacterial diarrhea, hepatitis A, and typhoid fever based primarily on patients' presenting histories and objective physical examination findings, I tried to get recipes for each in my mind. Other members of the team had been on these mission trips in the past; they knew the dearth of diagnostic testing available to corroborate history and physical examination data. To Rosa and me, our clinical skills were the primary tools available. I had graduated from UMDNJ with my post-master's certificate in 1998, and in 2001 I did not yet identify as an expert primary care provider. In fact, I thought my memo-writing skills as an administrator far exceeded my primary care skills. Rosa's presence was reassuring.

My interpreter, Speciose, a quiet, shy woman whose children had been hachetted to death in their classrooms during the 1994 genocide, remained at my side as I saw patients. Speciose and I developed a rhythm, and my confidence in my physical examination skills returned once I saw my first patient. Feeling comfortable again, as if I were back in the fast-track emergency department at University Hospital in Newark, but without the luxury of sophisticated equipment, I treated hundreds of patients, along with Rosa, primarily for infectious diseases and acute episodic problems. These villagers were lean, with lifestyles demanding walking, often over roughly etched dirt roads on circuitous ridges, with baskets balanced gingerly on their heads. Hypertension and cardiovascular disease, marks of affluent cultures, were virtually absent; lack of clean water, plumbing, screens for windows, and other engineering and public health matters were critical factors to the epidemiology of the diseases we treated.

HIV and AIDS—the thin man's disease—were common, with the country's overall life expectancy at forty-six years for both sexes, per World Health Organization data. Rosa and I regained confidence in, and respect for, the old-fashioned complete physical examination. I listened carefully to lung and heart sounds, examined wound drainage and urine for color and odor, teased out analyses of symptoms—or, chief complaints—to quickly run differential diagnoses in my mind. We frequently sought each other's counsel regarding the patients we saw. What we couldn't do was order chest X-rays, Magnetic Resonance Imaging (MRIs), Computerized Tomography (CT) scans, complete metabolic panels and cell counts through blood work, sonograms, echocardiograms, electrocardiograms, and other diagnostic tests that typically complete the database used to determine patients' differential diagnoses in the United States, at least for those with health insurance. The value of simply listening to patients was reaffirmed. Despite the obvious complexities of listening via an interpreter, patients' stories were important in Rwanda. Patient stories, or histories of the present illness, as these narratives are termed in the United States, gave us at least 50 percent of the clues; these clues then steered the physical examination, which focused patients' diagnoses and treatment. These are classic techniques that require two skills beyond those held by a practitioner: time and patience.

One patient, a young woman who appeared to be in her mid-to-late thirties, was brought to us by villagers. Speciose could not help me speak with her: she had little, if any, language skills. Known by villagers as the woman who lived alone on the mountain, she had been coaxed by neighboring villagers to come to the clinic for evaluation. When she was brought to my examination area, she backed into a corner, never taking her eyes off me, hunkered down on the floor, with a baby all the while breastfeeding. Scantily clad with a dingy T-shirt and a colorful skirt wrap, both malodorous and impregnated with dark reddish dirt, she presented with a large irregularly shaped mass in her mid-upper thorax; in fact, she had to lift the mass to allow the baby to breast-feed. She lived alone with her children in a mountain hovel. She had no language skills and shied away from my touch with both fear and repulsion. Here was Jodie Foster's 1994 *Nell*, with no possibility for a happy ending. She remained in the corner as other patients were cared for. As she watched me cautiously with patients, I imagined that she became comfortable, since she eventually allowed me to palpate the mass on her chest. She winced. I referred her to the physician on our team; he concurred that she would need a surgical evaluation, but that we had no such resource. Afraid to give her any medications, given that we could not adequately instruct her in safe usage, we simply requested the village nurses who had joined us to watch over her occasionally. We had hit a wall. Speciose suggested prayer.

I saw only one patient who starkly reminded me that I was in a postgenocide country, one still ravaged with hatred at the United Nations signage, cars, and representatives combing the landscape teasing out war criminals. A young Hutu male, carrying a rifle over his right shoulder and wearing the camouflaged uniform, army cap, and high-top boots of a soldier, entered my small corner of clinical space. As was always the case in University Hospital's emergency department, you get the next person in line when you are up for a new patient. Sometimes, given the luck of the draw, the next patient may be challenging, from any one of a number of perspectives. The rage and rebellion were familiar. The slung rifle was not. I was in Rwanda. With a sense of control over my clinical area, I told him, through Speciose, that he had to leave his rifle outside my area if he wanted to be evaluated. He complied. His chief complaint—at least the one he could voice for me to hear—was straightforward: a sexually transmitted infection. He was given antibiotics and instructions on the use of condoms. As he left, with the hint of a smile on his face as he primed himself for a photograph, I suspected that our instructions regarding condoms would go unheeded. In that violence against women commonly involved rape, condoms and all that they imply in U.S. culture—family planning and safety against infectious diseases—bore little value in this society. Why was I here? I recall looking at my teammates, including Speciose, and returned to my corner.

When we had completed our health services, we visited the medical university in Rwanda at its invitation. The dean there held a meeting for our team, inviting us to collaborate in enhancing the health services in Rwanda. Sitting at the head of a long conference table in a very warm, humid room immersed in sunlight streaming through broken windows rich with dirt, the dean sought us as partners to repair his population's health and to offer expertise and guidance

in establishing mental health services, physical therapy, knowledge of pros-
thetic devices, and an updated nursing curriculum. Other physicians were
also at the table, presumably medical school faculty. The building was old,
with an appearance of having been abandoned years earlier. Without resources,
paint was peeling off walls, and large, deep, pitted holes dotted the concrete
structures, the buildings dating from Belgium colonial days, absent the upkeep.
The dean sought an exchange of knowledge, with his faculty eager to learn
new skills; for nursing, the goal was clear—assistance to revise programming
to accommodate the needs of postgenocide communities. The goal was to get
knowledge, not material property. This request was clear and simple.

Upon my return to New Jersey, I submitted a report of my activities during
the trip to our university officials. While the chief of administration and finance
thought the request reasonable and responsible in a global society, others at
a central level and in the academic arm were not supportive. Claiming that
an expert in one of the medical schools had a program of research in a country neighboring Rwanda, a key administrator decided that cooperation with
the medical University of Rwanda's medical school would conflict with this
expert's work. Thus, the relationship I advocated was not to be.

This administrator's office had floor-to-ceiling bookshelves, a rich mahog-
any desk, luxurious couch and chairs, and elegant lamps. The air smelled
remarkably fresh, with excellent ventilation and air conditioning.

I left the office and resigned as dean.

When Is a Patient Encounter (Not) Complex?

When I first met Cynthia in fall 2010 at the Mary Howard Health Center in
Philadelphia, she entered my small but well-equipped examination room with
a full entourage, including a case manager and two medical students from the
University of Pennsylvania. After asking who the patient was, I dismissed the
two students, inviting them to continue their community outreach experience
in the waiting room. We were now down to a manageable threesome. When I
see patients with an escort, I wonder to myself why they can't be seen alone. Is
there a language issue? Is there a safety issue? Is the patient confused or not in
touch with reality? Is she hearing voices?

The Filipino case manager, Juan, introduced Cynthia to me, indicating that
she required a physical examination in order to remain at a sheltered residency
in North Philadelphia. Cynthia, a tall, thin, 160-pound, sixty-year-old African
American female, was beginning to have difficulties living in her home alone,
and she therefore fell within the protective services of the welfare system. Her
physical examination revealed a Body Mass Index of 24—normal weight for her

height—and Stage 2 hypertension. She had been treated for hypertension in the past, but she wasn't sure for how long she had been without antihypertensive medication. Her affect was absolutely flat, expressionless. No smile, no frown, but consistently responsive to questions; she also initiated conversation, asking me if we were about the same age. I told her that we were exactly the same age. She asked if I was careful with my bones. *Had I ever broken a bone?*

I told her that I was *scared to death of falling*, given my osteoporosis.

Did I hear voices also?

When I told her no, she volunteered that she did.

Do these voices ever tell you to hurt yourself or others? I asked.

No, she indicated; but she said she was amazed that we all asked that same question. *Do they teach you to ask this?* she pondered.

I asked her if she was willing to take two medications for her blood pressure—one a diuretic and the second a calcium channel blocker, both found to be particularly efficacious with African American patients.

How different are blacks and whites? she asked.

I assured her that *we are alike,* two sixty-year-old women, she with hypertension and hearing voices and me with osteoporosis and arthritis. She smiled.

We are alike, right? she asked shyly.

Yes, we are alike.

Juan took the prescriptions and we made appointments for a follow-up visit in one month and an urgent first visit with the psychiatric mental health nurse practitioner. We shook hands before she left.

When I saw Cynthia one month later, I was amazed at her weight loss—thirty pounds in one month, almost 20 percent of her previous weight—an ICD-9 code of 783.21. She has exceeded the criteria for unintentional weight loss as outlined for nursing home residents.

Do I have cancer? I must have cancer. I told her and Juan that her weight loss was quite stunning, and I agreed with her that cancer is a primary problem causing weight loss. But maybe we could think a bit more simply and eliminate other things first.

What was she eating at her new residency? Did she like the food? She told Juan to cover his ears, clearly afraid to hurt his feelings. *No,* she said, *I don't like their food. It's all carbs, most of the time,* she said. *When I have a few dollars,* she confirmed that she would *sneak a hot dog.* She loved these hot dogs! She had an appetite, but was not eating too much, given that she didn't like the food. She thought the food had no flavor; it was boring. And she was on so many medications that she was afraid that the food and the drugs might not be good together.

Can I stop some of the psych drugs? she asked, *I feel out of it most of the time now.*

I encouraged her to explore this option with her psychiatric nurse practitioner; I even invited her to negotiate down to one, two, or three drugs, rather than five.

When people think you are crazy, they act like you can't hear or think anymore, as if you couldn't make any decisions for yourself, Cynthia said. *You don't have any power when they think you're crazy,* she volunteered with passion.

I reassured her that it was *her* health and *her* illnesses and that *she* called the shots. To halt her weight loss, I encouraged her to eat as much as she wished to eat, all the hot dogs she could manage.

With a quick hug followed by a handshake, Cynthia walked out of the office. She got a third appointment for a follow-up visit in one month. Should I have given her prescriptions for complete blood work to rule out hyperthyroidism, diabetes, anemia, infection, malignancy, uremia, hypoproteinemia consistent with anorexia, or other diseases? Should her stool be tested for parasites and ova? A chest X-ray might reveal lung cancer, particularly relevant due to her past history of cigarette smoking. Colonoscopy? Endoscopy?

As I walked to the SEPTA subway that afternoon, I reviewed in my mind the common causes of unexplained weight loss, and compared these to Cynthia. She didn't like her present food, but she had an appetite. She was heavily medicated for psychiatric disorders, including depression, commonly associated with anorexia and weight loss. She had recently been relocated from her home to a transitional housing site, and thus no longer lived within her normal context. The array of possible diagnostic tests swirled around in my head. All I had done while she was in the office was a hemoglobin screening check for anemia; her test came back at the lowest limit of normal, 12. I determined to simply reevaluate her weight, hemoglobin, physical findings, and medications at our next visit. If needed, I would then send Cynthia for complete blood work, chest X-ray, urinalysis, and a screening colonoscopy. Based on these findings, we would determine the next steps.

I was overwhelmed by the complexity of this situation. I understood the context, and felt an appreciation for her living situation. I could envision Cynthia leaving the shelter, when no one was watching, and escape to the corner store where her favorite hot dogs were sold. After living in her own home for decades, she now sneaked hot dogs on the sly. Unlike the externalities of economics theory, all of Cynthia's context and story are critical to know and synthesize, if patient-centered health care management is to exist. Listen to the story and the context carefully; I know this is correct, but I still worry about what is considered "customary and usual" relative to this diagnosis. What would a jury of my peers have done for Cynthia the first time her weight loss was identified?

Margaret, in contrast to Cynthia, presented with an objective finding that typically warrants close examination. On her first visit, Margaret, deaf since childhood and proficient in signing with her partner—a man who consistently joins her in the examination room—presented with normal physical examination findings except for her hearing loss and tachycardia, a fast heart rate of 120 beats per minute. Since she was perimenopausal, excessive blood loss with menstruation may have been implicated; her hemoglobin, measured through Hemocue testing, was 11.5, below the normal. She was not on any medications and denied any use of recreational or street drugs. I gave her a prescription for complete blood work, in addition to a referral for hearing aids. When I saw her a month later and we looked at her electronic medical record together, it showed that I had ordered the blood work but it was not yet performed so results had not yet been received. Nor did she make an appointment to be evaluated for hearing aids. Since her partner was not with her on this repeat visit, Margaret and I wrote notes back and forth to each other. I had never learned sign language, nor Spanish, two skills truly vital in health care delivery.

She said firmly, with a calm resolution, that she would undergo the fingerstick in the office for hemoglobin testing, but would not undergo any other diagnostics or referrals. *I don't want these tests; I am OK without hearing aids*, she wrote, with a large smile on her face and her hand on my arm, reassuring me. Margaret's pulse on this second visit was now at 134 beats per minute; although she denied any of the usual symptoms associated with such severe tachycardia—chest discomfort or pain, shortness of breath, palpitations, fatigue, dizziness, weakness—I was really worried. Her hemoglobin had improved to 12.5 with her multivitamins-with-iron pills, no doubt, but she would not allow an electrocardiogram, blood work, or referrals. So we discussed diet, the signs that her tachycardia may be worsening, and what to do if she experienced chest pain or other severe cardiovascular or cerebrovascular complications. I had no reason to believe that she did not understand my rationale for further diagnostics; she simply refused to have them. I evaluated her as a reliable narrator and a patient competent to make decisions for herself. I remained uncomfortable when Margaret left the health center, with a follow-up appointment scheduled in one month. Was I overestimating her understanding of the consequences of unexplained tachycardia? Was I underestimating her deafness?

I documented the situation thoroughly in the medical record, conscious at the time that any record can be read in court. Patient-centered decision making is the core theme in what is now called the medical home; patients, simply put, call the shots. I had now felt the discomfort of primary care, with a patient for the first time simply telling me no, right at the beginning. Not a noncompliant patient, nor one that simply forgets. Rather, an informed decision maker, conscious and alert to consequences. Very disconcerting.

My experiences with Kyshan have been in the interstices between Cynthia and Margaret. Kyshan, a forty-two-year-old Hispanic male, was mugged in early fall 2010, with resultant injuries to his leg—a large laceration requiring suturing—and a blow to his left forearm immediately below his olecranon, the upper part of the ulnar bone. He was treated immediately after the trauma at his local emergency room and released. Told to visit his primary care provider, Kyshan came to me for a follow-up evaluation in early January 2011. The laceration on his leg had healed well, with very minor scarring. He continued to experience discomfort in his forearm, with weakness in lifting heavy objects and occasional numbness and pins-and-needles sensations in his arm, extending to his hand. He had trouble finding a good position for sleep, noting that he was now losing sleep and becoming fatigued in the daytime. I started with my standard treatment for musculoskeletal pain, nonsteroidal anti-inflammatory drugs (NSAIDs)—generic ibuprofen specifically. Although we discussed the need for progressive exercise of his left arm, including elbow flexion and extension, Kyshan was impatient, stating that he was too busy looking for a job to bother with exercises. He eagerly accepted the sample ibuprofens I gave him, and made another appointment for a follow-up visit. When he returned, he paced my small examination room, unable to sit down because he was angry that the ibuprofen didn't take away the pain, it only toned it down a little. He also said it felt like his bones were cracking against each other when he rotated his forearm at the elbow joint.

Since Kyshan had never had his left arm X-rayed, I wrote a prescriptions for an X-ray to rule out fracture and a different NSAID—Naproxyn. On his follow-up visit, he was increasingly angry. Naproxyn, like ibuprofen, was useless. And although he said he had the X-rays taken at a neighboring hospital, we had no report; and the hospital, when questioned, could not find any record of his visit. He then demanded Endocet, a generic form of Percocet, a combination drug of acetaminophen and oxycodone. An excellent drug to control pain, Endocet is a controlled dangerous substance with addiction potential. Rather than going down the path of prescribing Endocet for Kyshan, I asked him to sit and talk with me about his pain, his history of past addiction, and his honest plan for his future. He was visibly shocked when I explained that he might always have some discomfort related to his forearm injury. He might even have to learn to manage his pain with non-narcotics, exercise, and rest.

People live with pain? he asked. *Can they really manage their pain?*

We discussed a series of steps that he agreed to follow. First, get the X-ray; then, possible referral to neuro-orthopedics to evaluate his forearm and abnormal sensations—paresthesias; and finally, referral to pain management specialists to mutually develop a pain management regimen that would be effective for him, eventually one without narcotics. He left with another prescription for an X-ray and more samples of ibuprofen.

Cynthia, Margaret, and Kyshan were complex patients, with each involving decision making about need for further diagnostics and referrals to specialists. On a day when I am tired, or when the electronic medical record seems particularly slow or otherwise annoying, these types of complexities are very vexing. They involve real analyses of patients in their context and from their perspective; this type of analysis takes time, something not generally available in a managed care center. At Mary Howard, however, I usually have about a 50 percent no-show rate, which then reduces me to between four to five patients in the four hours I am there. On days with this type of patient load, I have the time to talk with patients. When demands for increasing productivity, as well as efforts at reducing no-show rates, are successful, then I will have less of that regaled commodity—time. If productivity rates do not increase, there will be more commodity than nurse.

Imperious Intellectus versus Accommodation Theory

Whether in the Camden community health center, Rwanda, or the Philadelphia's Mary Howard Health Center, I have often wondered why each patient visit takes me so long. Is it my inexperience, my lack of knowledge, my ineptness at the electronic medical record, or some other factors? Why do physicians seem to manage larger daily case loads than many nurse practitioners, including me? A closely associated question, one that has plagued me for years: What is the contribution of my nursing background to primary care delivery? A seemingly trite question. After all, I have been a registered nurse for decades; one would assume that I deeply appreciated nursing's contribution to primary care. Yet the nurse I once was is not the nurse I am now.

As I care for Cynthia, for example, I have begun to understand that I burden myself. I ask the next question. Cynthia lost weight, a significant loss in a short timeframe. *Are you eating?* I ask. Her answer: *No.* I then ask: *What is going on now that you don't eat?* It is the second question that embeds me in context, Cynthia's context. Having asked the question, I must now listen; I cannot ignore the wealth of information about her situation that illuminates her chief complaint: weight loss. Because Cynthia has Medicaid-managed care insurance, I could have ordered a variety of diagnostics (e.g., blood chemistries and other tests) immediately upon noting her weight loss. Instead, I listened. This took time. Together we decided to wait for a month before we ran additional tests. Should I eat more hot dogs? she asked. Absolutely, as many as you wish; plus, anything else you feel like eating, I advised. Cynthia has helped me understand nursing's contribution to primary care. I appreciate context—a nursing contextual knowledge as part of a management scheme.

Thus, context is a cornerstone construct in nursing, perhaps alluded to through different language. Knowledge of a patient's context makes or breaks a therapeutic plan. Why bother sending a patient home with multiple prescriptions if she has no means to pay for the medications and/or inadequate understanding of her drug regimens? Why instruct a battered woman on how to manage her lacerations and arm cast if she is simply discharged back to an abusive predator at home? While all providers, medicine and nursing alike, are intellectually aware that patients' environments deeply impact health—note that we all emphasize community and public health—and that management plans must be individualized to be effective, the use of context as a tool in the plan may not be addressed by both groups in the same way. How does a patient define his or her health? Do patients call the shots in their care? Or are they only there to rack as I cue?

During my early days at the University of Medicine and Dentistry of New Jersey, I gradually learned about the orientation of my colleagues in medicine. On a steamy hot day in August, I watched the White Coat ceremony of the New Jersey Medical School from the sidewalk at Twelfth and Bergen Streets. My hair felt plastered against my neck, a day when it was simply impossible to cool down, with no breeze wafting across the campus quad. A relatively new ritual in medicine, the White Coat ceremony marks the new students' entrance into medicine—a rite of passage akin to a priest's ordination to priesthood. Clearly, it is a transition marking entrance to a prestigious group, with public officials, Board of Trustees members, family and friends all in attendance. The message: you have entered the ranks of society's trusted elite. I recall my amazement. In my department, we had just begun a Doctor of Nursing Practice program, with no fanfare, no governor in attendance, only a mad scramble toward classrooms in the evening, when our students were off work and clinging to large cups of coffee in their hands as they came to class.

Inculcating prestige from day one, medicine marks their young as members of a group held in great esteem, at the pinnacle of U.S. society. Subliminal messages abound; medicine does not make mistakes, their young will succeed, their arrogance is justified, their costs necessarily passed onto others, others who should be grateful. The white coat symbolizes medicine. I now began to understand why I had had to battle a few years earlier at the Veterans Affairs Medical Center in East Orange, New Jersey. As their new patient education coordinator, with my gleaming new NYU PhD in hand, I was told that only physicians could wear white lab coats and only physicians could park in the doctor's lot. Intrinsically un-American. I fought, and won, parking privileges for PhD staff in the doctor's lot; but I did not win the battle for lab coats. I chose to wear street clothes in my role rather than a lab coat, a decision not appreciated by nursing administrators. In one moment, standing on the corner of Bergen and Twelfth Streets, I understood.

In the U.S. health care system, the physician is the lead player, directing the medical plan, instructing patients, their families, and other care providers about their roles: *imperious intellectus.* In the fabric of the lab coat is the faculty or ability to perceive the transcendent, the objectivity of *imperious intellectus.* Such ascribed capability carries with it ascendancy over those without such unique abilities. Physicians focus on the objectivity at hand, the data they see. Data in context is an externality, something for nursing to play with. Objective data are clean, at hand, and capable of management. Lawrence Weed's problem-oriented medical record, designed in the early 1970s, trained physicians to outline patients' medical problems based on data obtained through history (i.e., *S*ubjective data), physical examination (i.e., *O*bjective data), assessment (i.e., *A*ssessment or diagnosis), and medical plan (i.e., *P*lan). The acronym SOAP is now used by multiple health care providers in documenting patients' records. The extent to which a provider documents subjective findings is influenced by their professional perspective. In nursing, subjective data extend beyond the analysis of the patient's chief presenting complaint; it includes context. As context is examined, the provider invariably shares decision making with the patient. To exhibit willingness to know context is to be willing to negotiate or compromise with patients as to the therapeutic plan to be designed. If a patient is willing to accept medications to manage her hypertension, then which medications can she afford and which works well in her lifestyle? Maybe, as occurred with me in caring for Margaret, my patient with an extremely fast heart rate, a patient may not be willing to engage in the plan the provider advocates. My nursing perspective, threaded through my primary care practice, allows accommodation to my patients' situations. Nurses accommodate to situations at hand, including patient situations.

As health care reforms in the United States, a key debate continues around care delivered in medical-directed health homes versus patient-centered health homes. The *medical-directed* home is a team-based model of health care delivery in which the physician directs continuous primary care to patients with the goal of optimizing health outcomes. Nursing's model is that of a *patient-centered* health home, also a team-based model in which the patient is the center of decision making, with all providers coordinating quality service. The difference is essentially one of control: Will the physician design the plan of care, or will the patient direct such a plan? The National Committee for Quality Assurance (NCQA) is a private, nonprofit organization that accredits and certifies a wide range of health care organizations. In April 2011, the NCQA recognized fourteen federally qualified health centers as Patient-Centered Medical/Health Homes in Missouri and New York. A patient-centered medical home is an alternative to our fragmented delivery system, one in which patients are no longer silent partners in their care. As of 2011, nurse-managed health centers, under the clinical direction of a nurse practitioner, can achieve Level I Recognition by the NCQA, given compliance with at least five of the organization's ten elements. Without performance reporting by a physician, however, nurse-managed health centers cannot achieve Level 2 or Level 3 NCQA Recognition. Such recognition is critical to receiving reimbursement for health care services rendered.

Patient-centeredness is based on context; knowing context takes time. Time costs money. It is easier to base plans of care on objective data only, and then blame patients for noncompliance if such regimens fail. In context-framed care, noncompliance does not exist. An objective physician-based home may see more patients per day than a nurse-managed practice; thus, it may be applauded as a successful venture. The industry standard for the number of patients typically seen daily by one provider is about twenty. This is a soft standard, one that is more informal and customary than rigid. Most practices, based on context and preference as well as the need to make ends meet, sets an actual per day or per month goal for the number of patients they can see. Another standard that can be used is the Relative Value Unit (RVU)—a value that captures the level of time, skill, training, and intensity needed to provide a particular service. RVUs are used by Medicare, under the Center for Medicare and Medicaid Services, as a schema to determine how much money primary care providers should be paid for any particular service associated with a particular Current Procedural Terminology (CPT) code. The RVU methodology of reimbursement is controversial, with critics claiming it incentivizes specialty practice, since increased training is rewarded in the RVU formula. At the Mary Howard Health Center, the productivity standard was set at between ten and twelve patients per nurse practitioner daily in 2011.

In July 2010, I received a simple spreadsheet summary of productivity at the center. It included the monthly productivity goal of patients to be seen by each provider, the actual per day per month visits per provider, the over or under monthly goal figure per provider, and the actual year-to-date, over-or-under-goal figure per provider. On this sheet, my total monthly productivity goal was established at 12 patients; by the end of March 2011, my monthly goal had increased to 14, and my actual year-to-date had increased to 90 patients. My productivity was improving, with an actual per day per year now at 7.45 patients. (I find that 0.45 patient visit perplexing.)

Here thrive the aims of Frederick Winslow Taylor, the father of scientific management, a graduate of the Stevens Institute of Technology who developed time-and-motion studies to measure productivity. Several studies of nursing reported their findings in the early twentieth century; the Goldmark and Brown reports reviewed nursing education. Josephine Goldmark, a social scientist, noted in her 1923 report, *Nursing and Nursing Education in the United States*, that hospital service needs for workforce productivity jeopardized nursing education programs. The 1936 Brown report—*Nursing as a Profession*—was written by social anthropologist Esther Lucille Brown; it revealed that nursing students in hospitals continued to be used to meet workforce demands. How many patients can be cared for by nurses—or nursing students—during a shift? Similarly, patient care encounters drill down to widgets in an assembly line—how many widgets can be produced in a shift? The sheer reductionism of patient to widget, followed by revenue generation associated with the care of that widget, is an interesting hallmark of contemporary primary care delivery. I returned to my small corner of clinical space.

As an administrator, I deeply appreciated the urgency to generate patient revenue at the center. Simple math: more patients, more dollars. The center needed to generate enough revenue to pay not only for the nurse practitioner staff—both full time and part time—but also the medical assistants, scheduling clerks, referral clerk, and social worker. I became determined to produce error-free encounter forms. Errors on encounter forms delay billing insurers, which delay paying bills at the center. Encounter forms, listing correct CPT diagnostic codes and other billable items—such as blood work taken and other diagnostic tests performed—generate complete and accurate invoices. A perpetual student, I am competitive, particularly with myself, so I was horrified to learn that

I was not meeting the passing grade in the encounter form course. The clinical director reviewed the encounter form with me, reifying which boxes to check for both medical visits and family planning visits. A staff member was assigned to review my encounter forms before I put them in the biller's bin for the generation of invoices to insurers. I remediated, even purchased a book of ICD-9-CM codes and CPT codes as a reference. I placed a yellow sticky note on my computer screen, reminding me to review family planning with each patient: Have you asked about family planning today? The family planning encounter form is separate from the medical encounter form. On it, one documents birth control method used, types of counseling services provided, and diagnostic tests taken, with each item generating billable expenses. Since I routinely ask patients about their satisfaction with their sexual life and their method of birth control, I found it easy to place a large bowl of condoms and small paper bags on the corner of my desk. I began to offer all patients who expressed interest in sexual activity a bag of condoms at the end of each session. Most patients, I found, appreciated receiving this bag, some relieved of the burden of having to ask for them.

At one point, Temple University's Nancy Rothman complimented me on my progress with the family planning encounters; I had apparently improved in my family planning efforts. I felt good; my marks had improved. Nancy also reassured me that although she had been informed by the new billing professional at the Public Health Management Corporation—the owner of the Mary Howard Health Center—that the goal was for nurse practitioners to see about fifteen to twenty patients daily, she was advocating for less, given the complexity of the patients here. I was pleased to hear her say this. If the center switched from a ten patient per day expectation to a twenty per day model, I would have found a politically correct rationale for withdrawing my services. Perhaps the demands of our upcoming accreditation visit by the Collegiate Commission for Nursing Education warranted my increased attention; or, the college would no longer tolerate my volunteerism at the center, requiring me to resign unless payment for my services was provided. I would have devised an excuse. Sometimes I find myself discussing matters with my patients that are most paramount to them, but are clearly not medical diagnoses found in the CPT code book. A prescription with a referral to the Community College of Philadelphia for career advisement; or a patient-education discussion centered around management of a paternity suit; or a conversation about the values of employment versus public assistance. Some of my patients ask to return for follow-up on a monthly basis, simply to review, for example, their educational progress or to map out strategies on how to live "on the outside" of prison. These conversations are the essential gist of therapeutic lifestyle changes that are important to these patients. Without having time for these conversations, I would feel that I have cheated these homeless patients of beneficial health services.

In the April 23, 2011, *New York Times* story by Gardiner Harris about a solo family physician captured this complexity extremely well—*talking too much is the kind of thing that gets me behind*, a physician said, *but it's the only part of the job I like.* The extra time he spends talking with his patients has hurt his income. Time spent talking reduces the number of patients seen, and the reimbursements secured. As Harris documented, the transition to larger ambulatory practices with timed, focused encounters between patients and providers reflects current practice shifts. I love the challenge of differentially diagnosing patients' problems and then planning their care, but, like the family physician in the *New York Times* article, what I love most is my time talking with patients, learning their priorities and facilitating their decisions for leading quality lives. Medical diagnoses get patients in the door, conversations about their lives keeps them coming back. Most patients recognize the emergency rooms will manage their illnesses, and they use them freely for this purpose. It is the relationships that evolve that take on broader importance for improving health indices.

If You Get the Data, What Will You Do with It?

What do you make of these laboratory findings? asked my colleague Mary. Mary's patient, a forty-eight-year-old white male, was alert, oriented, and without any apparent sign of illness. His blood chemistry, however, was a stark contrast to his appearance. With almost every electrolyte value abnormal, as well as abnormalities in his values related to his kidney function, we were left asking: What was wrong with this picture? The patient was chronically homeless, having been denied a place in any city shelters due to his habitual infractions of rules. Diabetes insipidus? An occult oat cell cancer in the lungs presenting as diabetes insipidus? Or, could it be lab error? Mary decided to repeat the blood chemistry, wondering if the unusual pattern of abnormalities had righted itself during the time between the taking of the blood and the patient's follow-up visit. She also spoke with our collaborating physician, who provided simple advice: only ask for sodium and potassium levels rather than the complete panel. Don't ask for data that you will not be able to use in your management plan. Advocating a minimalist orientation, she advised against ordering diagnostic tests either because the patient had insurance—therefore why not order the test?—or because the provider wanted a full plate of data from which to make the differential diagnosis. My experiences in Rwanda, as well as in

Camden, had empowered me to be comfortable with listening to the patient's story and conducting thorough physical examinations. Armed only with a glucometer, a cholesterol screening tool, and a hemoglobin device in Camden, I had managed uninsured patients on the basis of my clinical skills and glucose, cholesterol, and hemoglobin values. Negotiations with patients about changes they were willing to make in their lifestyles complemented my tools, resulting in management plans surely deemed crude in our current health care system.

The pressure to order sophisticated diagnostic tests is burdensome. One Thursday afternoon, as I rushed to get to the health center by 1 P.M., a colleague followed me into my examination room, with a presence that made the little room feel suddenly like the dimensions of a shoebox. Her speech was urgent, her face only a few inches from my own. *I saw one of your patients yesterday*, she said. *Yes, how was he?* He complained of back pain and she ordered several diagnostic tests, including an MRI of his back to diagnose the cause of his pain. She was surprised that I had not ordered these tests previously. *Yes, it will be nice to have these results*, I volunteered, even if I disagreed with the need for them. Based on his story and my examination findings, I had diagnosed him with low back pain—or lumbago, ICD9 code 724.1—and my plan included nonsteroidal anti-inflammatory drugs (NSAIDs), rest, weight loss, and progressive exercise. He was also morbidly obese, with a BMI of 42.1, or World Health Organization class III obesity (BMI > 40.00). Obesity alone is a major risk factor of musculoskeletal pain, predominantly in the knee and lower back. While the tests my colleague ordered were appropriate, I simply disagreed with the need for them. The patient had not shown any sign of cauda equina syndrome, only positive straight leg raise tests.

My colleague was clearly pleased that she had managed this patient aggressively, my simple management plan seeming insufficient. For the rest of my afternoon I was a bit out-of-sorts. Intellectually, I knew that I would continue to manage this patient as I had previously, with a primary focus on weight loss, asking him to complete a diet diary at the end of each day that we would review together at each visit. The goal of a diet diary is to facilitate patient insight into dietary habits, helping him take the next step to eliminate certain foods in his diet over time. Emotionally, however, I was rattled and unable to concentrate. I practice one half-day each week, working in an office as an administrator for the rest of the week. While I keep up with clinical practice advances through continuing education, I was surprised that my colleague's aggressive management of my patient unnerved me so significantly. Did I lack confidence? Did she need to compete? Did she need to demonstrate her clinical superiority? Was I lax in collecting the necessary data to manage this man? Or was this just an example of nurses competing with each other, an extension of the phenomenon of nurses hurting their own? Even though his MRI result came back with only reports of osteoarthritic changes in his vertebrae, my discomfort lingered.

In a conference jointly sponsored by Temple's Department of Nursing and the Law School in spring 2011, panelists examined challenges in the U.S. health care delivery system. The medical director of Keystone Mercy Health Plan claimed that the game has been set against us for too long, with many tests too costly and ordered unnecessarily. Defensive medicine, with an overuse of diagnostic services, he claimed, has contributed significantly to the cost of health care. He advocated tort reform, along with calls for only medically necessary tests. Clearly, he is correct. But the context is much more complex than the simple statement implies. In cases when a patient claims malpractice on the part of a clinician, the question becomes: How would that clinician's peers have managed the case under similar circumstances? Did the patient's provider evidence any error of omission or commission? An act of omission is not conducting a test or procedure that may have led to an injury preventable by more optimal care. Did the provider forget to order a chest X-ray in a patient experiencing pneumonia but not diagnosed or treated thoroughly for this illness? Or, did the provider demonstrate an act of commission? That is, did the provider conduct a task incorrectly? Or, did the provider plan care incorrectly or execute a management plan improperly? Medical liability claims in the United States were roughly 10 percent of all tort litigation in 2008, with most costs attendant to legal costs rather than patient compensation, as noted by Amy Lynn Sorrel in her May 2, 2010, article "Medical Liability: A World of Difference" in the *American Medical News.* How much data is enough to collect? Is the data really necessary to determine a patient management plan?

Once you get the data, what will you do with it? Providers define the phrase "medically necessary" quite differently in practice. If a patient presents with health insurance and a legitimate medical diagnosis—low back pain— then diagnostic tests may be approved by the insurer. But are those tests really needed? Providers confident in their physical examination skills and ability to differentially diagnose may not be confident that their peers would agree with their management. Bottom line: it is less risky to order more diagnostic tests than fewer tests. Although additional tests may inconvenience patients (and worry them unnecessarily) and increase overall costs to the system, risks to providers decrease. Pneumonia can be diagnosed on the basis of history and physical examination findings; chest X-ray, however, continues to be the gold standard for the diagnosis of pneumonia and to identify complications. With an increasing arsenal of clinical experience, confidence also expands, and perhaps less reliance on costly diagnostic tests to substantiate clinical diagnoses. The lingering cloud of liability—and the jury of peers—looms over practice, making you question your actions.

When my sixty-year-old patient Cynthia presented for a follow-up visit to evaluate her weight loss, she had now lost an additional 3 pounds—a total of 33 pounds in just eight weeks. Yes, she had been eating a bit more, and yes, her appetite for hot dogs was great. I now followed the protocol outlined in *Harrison's Principles of Internal Medicine*—I ordered a full panel of blood work, chest X-ray, a 12-lead electrocardiogram (her heart rate was 99/minute), and a screening colonoscopy. I knew that Cynthia would have these tests done; she and Juan, her case manager, would make the appointments themselves and we three would review the results when they were available. I left the health center that evening feeling confident that these tests were warranted and appropriate.

As I walked west on Sansom Street to reach the SEPTA station, I thought of my daughter in Florida who had an appointment with a neurologist that day to evaluate her headaches. A thirty-two-year-old reading teacher in a public school in Boca Raton, she had a history of chronic upper respiratory infections, migraine headaches, seasonal allergies, and an on-again, off-again history of cigarette smoking. When initially evaluated by her primary care physician, she was treated with antihistamines, nasal corticosteroids, and a course of antibiotics. When reevaluated, she was referred for MRI evaluation of her sinuses. The results were negative; subsequently, she was referred to a neurologist to confirm a rule-out diagnosis of migraine headaches. Based on her description of her headaches, the neurologist confirmed migraine headaches and prescribed a triptan for management, a very common drug treatment. To be safe, however, given my history of a presumed arteriovenous malformation in my brain which resulted in a bleed, he also ordered an MRI of her brain. If negative, this test would give her important information, and a baseline for further evaluation in the future.

I sat in my favorite seat on the train, the one in the very first car next to the driver. From this seat I could watch us rumble along quickly past the graffiti-painted walls from station to station. As I sat, drained and eager to return to South Jersey, a large muscular man, dressed with a religious collar and a white suit, began preaching in my car. Absolutely no one attended to him. I got off at my usual stop—Allegheny Street—on the Temple University Health Sciences Campus. Through cold drizzling rain at 7 P.M., I walked past our dental school to approach the parking garage. Two morbidly obese physical plant workers exited the dental school, pushing a cart carrying food trays and soda cans, probably on their way to, or from, a school event. In April, schools hold celebrations to honor graduating students and their families. I was impressed by their obesity, their exceptionally slow, lumbering gait, and their breathlessness. I passed them quickly and walked beyond them toward the local barbershop, a popular hangout in the neighborhood. Located as a split-level structure, with a staircase going below ground, this shop was a local haunt. Street vendors propped up their wares adjacent to the shop, and panhandlers lined the walls of the shop, all welcomed. Next to this shop, a Dunkin' Donuts, and then a liquor store. A vibrant area, it often seemed like a prop for a movie scene designed to titillate suburban audiences with scenes of colorful urban squalor. I was also a familiar figure, given my daily walk to and from the subway station. Heads nodded as I passed. That evening, thinking of my daughter as I walked past this familiar area, I was struck by the contrast of these residents' lives with my own.

I have sometimes characterized certain aspects of health care delivery in cities as the "middle earth" of our system, capitalizing on J.R.R. Tolkien's *Lord of the Rings.* The Hobbits, notably Bilbo Baggins and his cousin Frodo Baggins, are sent on a mission to retrieve the One Ring, the ring with ascendant power. The city's rich network of community-based services, including the nurse-managed health centers (such as Mary Howard) provide a safety net for many of the residents I pass daily on the streets of North Philadelphia. I am a Hobbit of health care close to the ground.

While the system of care provided to city residents in poor neighborhoods is less visible than that found in ambulatory practices within more affluent communities, it nevertheless provides full services, including referrals to specialists. Whether receiving Medicaid managed care or care managed by a third-party insurer, the urge to order excessive diagnostic tests prevails. There is worry over malpractice liability claims, as well as the need to rely on diagnostic test data in lieu of time spent listening to, and physically examining, patients. As the conveyor belt of managed care moves patients along at fifteen- to twenty-minute intervals, time is saved on listening and examining. Data, therefore, must be obtained by taking the more expensive route—additional testing.

I hope that Nancy is right and that the health center will not increase patient visits to twenty per provider per day. At times, I explore alternative models in my mind, afraid to explore them openly. If nurse practitioners receive 85 percent of the reimbursement provided to physicians for the same service, then would it be more profitable to staff the health center with one or two physicians and less costly medical assistants than four nurse practitioners? It would mean higher reimbursement and perhaps more patients seen daily. The answer is to be found in the broad tundra between *imperious intellectus* and accommodation. I want to have time to write my message on a prescription: See an advisor at the Community College of Philadelphia.

If You Don't Write It, You Didn't Do It

In the early 1980s, as a young assistant professor of nursing at Rutgers University College of Nursing in Newark, New Jersey, I jockeyed my way among the faculty of the Acute Care Department to secure a plumb clinical site for my senior baccalaureate students—the Medical Intensive Care Unit (MICU) in the University Hospital of the University of Medicine and Dentistry of New Jersey. As an intensive care nurse certified by the American Association of Critical Care Nurses, I was ecstatic about my coup. As a young nursing intensivist with a long ponytail and crisp white lab coat, pockets spilling over with notebooks and equipment, I planned a clinical rotation for my students that would truly be a capstone experience—learning medical-surgical nursing in an environment where the sickest patients were cared for by stellar nursing and medical professionals. We would have nine students in an intensive clinical setting, all within an academic health center environment, a milieu of interdisciplinary colleagueship. Going into the semester, I anticipated a positive, stunning experience for my students.

The first day in the MICU, the chief medical resident asked if my students know how to measure urine. I was taken aback. Surely he jests? Surprisingly, he was serious. Over several clinical days, my negative experiences accumulated more quickly than my positive ones. Could my students run blood to the lab? Could they do patients' bed baths? Yes, they could do all of these things, as could others on staff. My goal, however, was for them to engage in nursing management of critically ill patients. I found myself competing with medicine for my students to perform certain interventions—changing complex dressings, managing invasive lines used to measure critical parameters such as atrial pressures and venous pressures, and more. I slowly came to see the disadvantages of teaching nursing within an academic health center setting. Everyone competes for experiences; medicine always wins. The academic health center hierarchy informally, and powerfully, establishes a clinical education caste system within which patients exist as cannon fodder for the education of medicine's young. Nursing students, the Dalits of the health care system, skirt the parameters by doing the tasks of the untouchables. I was young, and discouraged, but astute enough to recognize the value of the MICU for students to appreciate the care required of critically ill patients.

As I learned to make peace with the complexities of the MICU, I aggressively pursued a path for my students that I thought critical—documentation on the patient's medical record. If you didn't write it, then you didn't do it—an old adage made real by finding yourself as a defendant in court. You say you called the attending physician, but where in the medical record did you document that you called him? Your license is at risk without documentation. Documenting patient care is a complex venture, one requiring command of a common, shared lexicon. Prior to my faculty appointment at Rutgers University, I had worked as a staff nurse in the MICU of the Veterans Affairs Medical Center (VAMC), East Orange, New Jersey. At the VAMC, I became an advocate of Lawrence Weed's Problem-Oriented Medical Record (POMR) system of documentation. The POMR system organized patient information around patients' problems, with all subjective data, objective data, assessment, and plans linked to specific problems. As a problem resolved, it was retired; active problems were managed by health care providers with each participating according to his or her specialty knowledge. One record per patient; one charting system derived from the patient's problems, with all providers—physicians, nurses, social workers, others—working off the one POMR. When introduced in 1969 by Lawrence Weed, documentation revolutionized. Gone was the patient chart with separate tabs for each provider group to document within—nurses' notes, physician's notes, and others. Even the tab sections in the paper record reflected the implicit hierarchy: physician notes at the beginning of the record, nurses' notes at the end.

The POMR method shifted focus to the patient: What were the patient's problems? In my VAMC days of the early 1970s, I documented my care in the provider notes, along with all of my colleagues. My notes might precede or follow the physician's last entry; the system was egalitarian, with the advantage that different providers might actually read the previous note written by someone outside their field. It was an attack on disciplines' incestuous behaviors. At that time, the practice of charting by exception gained followers, a system of charting explained by Laura J. Burke and Judith A. Murphy in their 1995 book *Charting by Exception Applications: Making It Work in Clinical Settings* that was designed to minimize clerical activities; notations were to be made only when deviations from baseline or expected outcomes occur.

I loved Weed's POMR. Clean, simple, focused on the patient. And, not insignificant, it was interdisciplinary charting. It sharpened providers' clinical thinking, asking them to differentiate between subjective data—what the patient says, what he/she complains of—and objective data—physical examination findings, diagnostic data, referral findings. Since my very first experiences in charting under the section labeled *Nurses' Notes* in patients' records, I abhorred the language used. Patient appears lethargic, poor appetite, visitors at bedside, up ad lib to bathroom, and oriented X 3. Vague, useless, not worth the paper the notes were written on. Professionally embarrassing. Given my indoctrination to the POMR at the VAMC, I enthusiastically had my senior Rutgers nursing students chart in the physicians' notes at University Hospital, since they continued to have a separate tab for nurses' notes. In that it was highly unlikely that anyone would read their notes if placed in the nurses' notes section, I had them document their findings in the physicians' section using the POMR method. I had found this method a valuable educational tool, one that facilitated clinical reasoning, particularly in documenting histories and physical examination findings. One afternoon, the MICU resident read my student's neurological assessment findings of a patient recently admitted. He was impressed with the documentation, but quite upset that she had written her notes in the physician's section. *Would you have read her notes if they had been written in the nurses' notes section?* I asked. *No,* he said. *Her notes, however, were valuable in understanding the patient's neurological status, correct?* I asked. *Yes,* he indicated, *but she didn't have the right to chart in the physician's section of the medical record.* An incident evolved; the nurse manager instructed me to only chart in the nurses' notes section. But no one reads nurses' notes!

The next day I removed my students from the MICU and continued our clinical rotation in another, nonacademic health center hospital in Newark.

Beyond where one documents, the matter of what one documents also illustrates power. Crossing the Rubicon, nurses began a struggle to employ the language symbolic of medicine's power in the 1970s. Diagnosing and treating versus following orders and caring for patients; physicians' ownership of patients versus nurses' subservience to medicine. He who owned the word diagnosis had control, and ultimately, reimbursement. In 1991, nurse practitioners in New Jersey were defined by law as primary care providers, holding prescriptive authority; this same privilege was earned in Pennsylvania in 2002.

As a nurse practitioner in the Community Health Center in Camden, New Jersey, I was a solo provider, caring for uninsured and underinsured patients in the local neighborhood. I was busy. With a small interest account from an endowment to the center, I purchased a large, four-drawer, horizontal file cabinet to store paper medical records. While we had a graduate nursing informatics program at the University of Medicine and Dentistry of New Jersey, I was amazingly unsuccessful in designing and implementing an electronic system of charting medical records. The center was in an old building with poor wiring; the informatics faculty was not interested in this electronic record initiative. With multiple people on the one computer at the center, it more often than not was down with viruses, sick and ready to crash just as you would enter patient data if such medical record software were installed. I invariably left my charting to the end of the day. My scribbled notes on a small spiral notepad were my only means of recalling each patient. I then designed my standard medical record, a version of charting by exception; a four-page record for documenting a complete history and physical examination as well as an acute episodic note. Using the information published in *Barbara Bates' Guide to Physical Examination*, I created a template for normal findings for each body system, with a small area to document any exceptions. I photocopied this document and filed it in my top desk drawer in the examination room. It saved me! I used it routinely, feeling confident that I could defend my diagnoses and treatment plans based on my documentation. After eight hours in the health center, I finally left in a timely manner, my records complete. Thirty years into nursing, I had finally solved charting in this small primary care site.

While pleased with my documentation template, the age of electronics in the twenty-first century injected new hope that charting would not only be streamlined but also a source of data mining in evidence-based research projects. If records were stored electronically and universally accessible by appropriate providers, then one could address such questions as: What is the relationship of diabetes education on patient outcomes, including, for example, the hemoglobin A1c value? How many patients with asthma were treated in emergency departments in the last month? What is the relationship between home management regimes for congestive heart failure patients to episodes of acute pulmonary edema? Electronically accessible records eliminate tabs for notes written by different providers in a paper record; notes by all providers are visible to all who have access to records. As with online education through platforms such as Blackboard, electronic medical records transform documentation. Templates taken to the tenth power! Passage of Public Law 111–148—Patient Protection and Affordable Care Act—addresses the need for use of an electronic health record that would be universally available to all providers, eliminating redundancy in records management and enabling rapid retrieval of information when needed. Prior to this act, the Medicare Improvements for Patients and Providers Act of 2008 (MIPPA) included mandates to increase electronic prescribing (e-prescribing). In fact, nurse practitioners who do not e-prescribe or properly document e-prescriptions can be penalized with Medicare cuts in 2012, as noted in the minutes of the April 20, 2011, meeting of the Pennsylvania Coalition of Nurse Practitioners Philadelphia Chapter.

As I began my practice at the Mary Howard Health Center after I joined Temple University in 2008, I was trained for three hours in the use of the electronic medical record used by the Public Health Management Corporation (PHMC) at all of their nurse-managed health centers. I found it exciting. Click and send. The promise of efficiency and accuracy; no more staying late to finish patients' records! I was surprised to find the system a bit challenging, however. I blamed my ineptness on my part-time status. I found myself having to stay behind to complete my electronic records after seeing my patients. As with e-learning systems, the sheer visibility of my entries gave me pause. What was the best word or phrase to use? Did my physical examination findings adequately justify my diagnoses as entered on the encounter form? Did my physical examination findings and diagnoses justify further diagnostics and referrals? Despite my love of e-learning technologies, I found myself, at least in my early use of the electronic medical record (EMR), to be scrolling down to infinity to find the best word to describe, for example, the abnormal sounds I heard in patient's lungs. I wanted to click on "crackles," but the closest choice available was rhonchi. And, yes, I could write in the word crackles, but this seemed to obviate the need for an efficient clicking system. Although I fought against it, I found myself dreading the point when I had to chart using the EMR at the end of my clinical day.

My efficiency improved over time. At one point I brought in my paper document created for use at the Camden Community Health Center. I placed it on my desk next to the computer, and I frequently used the language on it when documenting on the EMR. For each body system for the physical examination, there is an icon of a pencil in the EMR. Clicking on this icon enables the provider to write comments freehand. When I mentioned this to a colleague who worked at another center, she urged me to create my own template and to have it stored under my name on the electronic system. Ta-dah! An intersection of my comfortable former system with the new EMR. True progress. As I stayed behind on my clinical day to chart on the EMR, I realized that I was not alone. Most nurse practitioners at the center were also still in their exam rooms, doors closed, frantic about completing their record entries. One would occasionally leave shortly after seeing her patients for the day, but spend hours at home completing her documentation on her personal computer, since the software application could be entered from a remote connection. While I do not abhor the EMR, I do admit to seeing it simply as an alternate way to document on the patient's record. Clearly, the advantages for universal access among providers, data mining, and accuracy for billing make the EMR exciting. At 7 P.M. on a February evening, when you had hoped to be home much earlier, the EMR simply becomes a provider's burden, as was its predecessor the paper record in another century.

One day, the computers were down at Mary Howard. We were forced to use paper records that day. We completed our work in a timely manner and got out at a reasonable time. Progress can indeed be painful to the individual provider. Many of us slugged home where men and children nested in couches, waiting.

Value Dualism and the Good Doctor

After six months of planning, an interdisciplinary group of nursing and law faculty at Temple University held a conference in April 2011 called "Beyond Paradigm Shift: Primary Health Care in a Post-Reform Period." It was a large success—over one hundred nurses and lawyers attended. On a lovely Friday afternoon in spring, I found myself intrigued by the enthusiasm and practical knowledge of one panel speaker, Eric Berman, an osteopathic physician educated at the University of Medicine and Dentistry of New Jersey's School of Osteopathic Medicine in Stratford. As the chief medical officer for Keystone Mercy Health Plan, Eric spoke to the need for productive primary care providers, including nurse practitioners. During the afternoon break, I introduced myself to him. He asked what programs in nursing we offered at Temple. I mentioned the adult and family primary care nurse practitioner programs, offered in a Doctor of Nursing Practice (DNP) program. *A clinical doctoral program for nurse practitioners?* he asked, a quizzical expression on his face. *A terrible development*, he proclaimed. *Nurse practitioners are midlevel providers, less expensive than a physician*, he said, adding that *now you will want more money because of the doctorate. Doctor nurse.* He shook his head, but left only after I secured a date to discuss this matter in more detail with him.

I arrived at the headquarters of the Keystone Mercy Health Plan headquarters early on a Monday afternoon in May. Centrally located within the environs of the Philadelphia International Airport, the four-story newly constructed building was impressive. A city person forever vigilant about parking, I found a spacious visitors' parking lot, inclusive of freshly mulched flowerbeds and devoid of hostile signage threatening your life if your car was left for more than twenty minutes. I found a spot easily, quite close to the main entrance. Very welcoming, even gracious. The main lobby was impeccably clean, with a waiting area complete with plush, comfortable chairs and end tables. To my left people were going in and out of a Federal Reserve credit union office; to my right, the Keystone Court Café was busy closing down operations for the day. My visitor pass was quite formal, with my name imprinted on it; I was instructed to wear it at all times while in the building. The lobby security officer who gave me my badge called Eric's office to let his staff know that I had arrived. *Someone will come down for you shortly*, I was informed. I waited by the café, intrigued by the comings and goings at the secure turnstiles—employees swiping their identification cards to gain access electronically. Always fascinated by people, I looked at the employees as they came or went, appreciating that the collective body mass indices (BMIs) of those I saw were in the overweight or obese categories. In general, unhealthy; as BMI increases, so too does risk for diabetes mellitus, hypertension, hypercholesterolemia, and cerebrovascular disease. Such a visible health problem. I was reminded of Michelle Obama's *Let's Move!* campaign to combat childhood obesity. As the First Lady had said in an interview on *Good Morning America* in February 2010, "We want to eliminate this problem of childhood obesity in a generation." As I casually looked at the Keystone staff angling to pass through the electronic gatekeepers, I thought to myself that we are certainly losing this battle with adults.

Two professional staff members met me in the lobby and escorted me to Eric's office. Both registered nurses, they were involved in quality initiatives at Keystone and very supportive of nurse practitioners. All four of us participated in a discussion on nurse practitioners, primary care providers, and issues such as productivity standards. Keystone Mercy Health Plan had identified nurse practitioners as primary care providers (PCPs) as early as ten years ago, Eric indicated. Why did Keystone, a Medicaid health plan, identify nurse practitioners as PCPs? The simple answer: cost. Lower cost and good outcomes. Nurse practitioners, according to Eric, are effective in providing outreach, educating patients in disease management, and performing interventions that physicians have neither the training nor time to do effectively. Bottom line: nurse practitioners can do basic primary care and they communicate much better than physicians. As to why nurse practitioners receive only 85 percent reimbursement compared to the 100 percent received by physicians for the same service, Eric agreed that this difference was directly related to relative value units—value units for work performed, practice expense, and malpractice—as well as the geographic practice cost index. Eric adamantly exclaimed that *nurse practitioners are missing the boat! Where were nurse practitioners going when they raised the educational standards to a clinical doctorate? They will blur the lines between physicians and nurse practitioners, much as physical therapists have done when they mandated a clinical doctoral degree for entry into practice. Nurse practitioners do not have the clinical knowledge of physicians, and yet they want patients to call them doctors!*

Physicians, Eric said, see one patient every eight minutes; he stated that he usually manages forty to forty-five patients in a day. He claimed that the eight minutes-per-patient ratio was an industry standard. In a six-hour clinical day, Eric's math is correct—eight minutes per patient, or forty-five patients per six-hour clinical day. Nurse practitioners, in contrast, see fewer patients, given that they provide more education. However, he was appalled when I told him that the expectation at the Mary Howard Health Center was twelve or more patients per day. *That is just not productive enough*, he exclaimed. *What happened during the eight minutes of your visits?* I queried. Management of the patients' acute episodic illnesses—the sore throat, the recurrent headache, the urinary tract infection—or monitoring of their chronic illnesses, such as reviewing insulin regimens for a diabetic patient. I thought of Donald Parks, one of our collaborating physicians for the nurse practitioners working at nurse-managed health centers in Philadelphia. He had advised that nurse practitioners must focus on the single most pressing chief complaint during a visit. Focus and, subsequently, control the visit to manage the primary presenting problem. Eric understood that nurse practitioners provided a more personal touch, communication being a strong suit for nurses in general. He stressed that nurse practitioners will be viable as PCPs as long as they keep their education realistic—*no need*, as he said, *for a clinical doctorate with just a lot more courses like English!*—and their costs down. A hidden cost to physicians, he explained, was the need for physicians to sign collaborative practice agreements with nurse practitioners, something akin to a travesty. *How much would I charge per month*, he hypothesized, *to serve as the collaborating physician for a nurse practitioner?* Given what he perceived to be the malpractice liability associated with such agreements, he was uncertain as to the fee he would charge. While liability and risk would be assumed by nurse practitioners in collaborative agreements, physicians would be responsible for the terms of the agreement they accepted, along with the fee provided. Mixing a modern worldview of medicine with a postmodern global need for expanded primary care causes clashes at the intersections of care with risk, and care with finances.

Conversing with Eric on the role of the generalist-practice registered nurse was equally illuminating, in that I glimpsed at a broadly held view that formal higher education was unnecessary for nurses. In advocating that baccalaureate-educated registered nurses (RNs) were best prepared to manage patient education regimens to prevent complications, reduce expensive hospital admissions, and eliminate associated co-morbid costs, I found Eric's and his two nursing colleagues' opinions to be radically different. *Why*, questioned Eric, *would we expose patients to "à la carte" medicine?* First, a patient visits the PCP for diagnosis and management of diabetes, for example. Subsequently, would the patient schedule a visit with the RN to learn diabetes self-management, insulin preparation and injection techniques, etc.? I argued *yes*, that *education is a reimbursable intervention*, one with evidence to support it as a separate billable item—billable to the RN who provided the service. Eric, however, mounted another approach; that is, code the encounter at a higher complexity level and check off all of the V codes as applicable to the patient. Thus, the reimbursement, based on the complexity level of the visit, will be supplemented by the V codes identified by the PCP and acknowledged in the bill submitted to the insurance provider. It is an interesting alternative, one that retains medicine's modernistic worldview, simultaneously assuring that all other potentially reimbursable services to nonphysicians continue to be bundled under the PCP's level of charted complexity. It is also a paternalistic view, one that secures medicine's controlling hierarchy, an enigma in the face of mounting evidence-based research on shared decision making and the country's demands for removal of barriers for full-scope practice for nurse practitioners.

As I dropped off my identification tag and returned to my car, I wondered: Can medicine succeed in retaining the old world structure of the failing health care system, simply because of wealth and power? Hallmarks of wealth are everywhere, from the café to the glossy publications on end tables, from the willing assent of Eric's nurses to his denial of the need for further education for registered nurses—evidence of a pre-health care reform era. In this gleaming world, the question had been asked and answered with the solid affirmation that accompanies power. Pennsylvania, as of 2011, had 7,298 certified nurse practitioners of which only 4,844 (or 66%) have prescriptive authority. Public Law 111–148—the Affordable Care Act—describes a new entity, the Accountable Care Organization (ACO), in section 3022, as a program that promotes accountability for a patient population, employing "redesigned" care processes. To be designated an ACO, the program must be willing to be accountable for the quality, cost, and overall care of the beneficiaries assigned to it. Under the Affordable Care Act, primary care providers were defined as physicians, osteopaths, and nurse practitioners. Under proposed rules published in the Federal Register in April 2011, nurse practitioners were excluded in a crucial section—D. Assignment of Medicare Fee-for-Service Beneficiaries—that states that assignment to ACOs is to be determined on the basis of primary care services provided by ACO professionals who are physicians. This proposed rule obfuscates an original intent of Public Law 111–148: to expand primary care services to those Americans currently uninsured or underinsured. To do so, nurse practitioners must expand their services—and their numbers—to fulfill the intent of the law. Quite surreptitiously, this proposed rule to return to medicine's hierarchical model both assures continuation of the country's illness focus as well as medicine's control over reimbursement.

With the language of ACOs also come terms such as medical home, patient-centered medical home (PCMH), or client health home. A "medical home" is a practice location where care for patients is coordinated among various health care providers—a "one-stop shop" for health management. With Public Law 111–148 using this language, the question has become: Can nurses, or nurse practitioners, lead PCMHs? The National Committee for Quality Assurance (NCQA) defines a PCMH as a model in which episodic care is replaced with coordinated care and a long-term relationship between the patient and the provider. The NCQA managed this politically volatile issue by use of the term "primary care clinician" rather than the older "primary care physician," making this change in fall 2010. Thus, NCQA has battled for PCMH with primary care clinicians, including nurse practitioners as lead agents, for several years. At a grassroots level, nurse practitioners have enjoyed new roles in many states, with even the popular press acknowledging the need to expand scopes of practice for RNs as well as nurse practitioners. Medical model versus health care model. If one only has eight minutes to manage a patient, then the only item managed is the chief presenting complaint—that is, illness care. If one dares to ask a patient how he or she is feeling generally, or if he or she has any other questions, or if preventive health questions are explored (for example, pneumonia immunizations for the elderly, HIV testing for those at risk, or questions regarding mental health, use of alcohol or other substances), then ten minutes have already passed and a stethoscope has not yet even been placed on the patient's chest. As the clock on the wall of the Mary Howard Health Center ticks closer to 5 P.M., I find myself switching from a health model to a medical model, simply due to time constraints. It is easier to manage acute illness than to manage health. As my colleague Carolyn, who works at an American Indian Health Center in Kansas, states, *these patients are complex—they take time!* Visits by complex homeless patients, like Carolyn's Indian patients, take time if the goal is to improve their health status. Fighting for a health model rather than an illness model through issues such as patient-centered medical homes, versus medical homes and through definitions of primary care providers for ACOs is time-consuming, requiring a vigilance that is exhausting. Such vigilance mandates resources, including lobbying for language change, and subsequently, reimbursement. As Betsy Snook, chief executive officer for the Pennsylvania State Nurses Association, said as the debate over leadership of ACOs raged, *the American Nurses Association was working to modify the language to make it more inclusive of other providers.* Does nursing have adequate staff and lobbyists to ensure adequate vigilance? I recalled a note that Stanley Bergen, president of the University of Medicine and Dentistry of New Jersey, had written on the back of a card included in a bouquet of roses that was sent to me by my dean colleagues in 1990: *Remember that the snakes are still in the grass!*

As I review my e-mails from colleagues regarding debates about medical homes and ACO leadership, a note comes in from one of my patients at Mary Howard, a forty-eight-year-old male with hypertension, hypercholesterolemia, and renal disease.

He wrote: *I was told from keystonemercy I need to look into ACEI_ARB THERAPY CAD and Antiplatement THERAPY CAD what is that thay it show I need to get check for that pleas let me know whats going on thank u.*

I called him, inviting him to come to see me as soon as possible, that we would discuss what CAD meant, and what the indications were of the other drugs this insurance provider mentioned. I also asked him to bring in the letter from the provider. I look forward to seeing him and to discussing his concerns with him. I also asked him to try to get my last appointment on a Thursday, ensuring that we could take time to talk—this would be more than an eight-minute visit. With its focus on healthy lifestyles, primary care is a time-consuming venture. This patient was a student at a local workforce development program, with access to computers and e-mail. This access opened a door to knowledge for him, just as my more educated and affluent colleague in Cambridge, Massachusetts, surfs the internet for current evidence-based practices in atrial fibrillation management.

In the digital world, dualisms of hierarchies, both oppressive and costly, dissolve.

Chapter 6

Barriers, Opportunities, and Militancy

Militants act, so says Antonio Gramsci. Nursing's history is resplendent with studies of the future of nursing. Authored by non-nurses claiming interest in the public's welfare, these reports rob nurses of their very voices. The most recent such report, published in 2011 by the Institute of Medicine in cooperation with the Robert Wood Johnson Foundation, identifies recommendations to be implemented in states through multidisciplinary action coalitions. Well-meaning as it may be, the report is nevertheless a litany, the tyranny of the *shoulds*, composed by non-nurses and tossed to nurses to implement. My experiences in post-riot Newark in the late 1960s illustrate that action by militants stimulates change. Appreciating the consequences of unhealthy lifestyles at the street level, my time as an academic administrator was often best spent on moving educational programs beyond hospitals into neighborhood health centers where nurses could advocate for healthy lifestyles. Given regulations by state boards of nursing mandating that nurse practitioners provide primary care through collaboration with physicians, the resulting litany of medical power, money, and greed frequently stalls such local nurse alternatives in urban areas marked by poverty. Identifiable barriers to nurse practitioner practice, couched in language ostensibly supporting quality care delivery, have been formally erected (restriction on scope of practice codified in law and regulations) and informally practiced (medical hierarchy built on attendant nurse subservience). Tacit barriers have subsequently fuelled nursing's failure to thrive. The academy shuns nursing faculty practice plans, and philanthropic foundations fail to support bold nursing initiatives. Leading to action, militancy must disrupt these barriers, set to deny health care as a basic human right. My experiences with authentic leaders have helped me understand that disruption is the order of the day; together, my colleagues and I have reimagined the reimbursement system to an HIV/AIDS facility, created an urban safety net system in several inner cities overwhelmed by poverty, and advanced agendas in which nurses lead nursing. In retirement, I look forward. Militants act, so say I. So say we all.

*

From my recliner chair facing the head of Miss Millie's bed, I anticipated that her twenty-second apneic period would be followed by a pattern of crescendo-decrescendo alteration in tidal volume—Cheyne-Stokes breathing, a pattern of breathing often noted in those with severe cerebral brain injury. As her respiratory depth increased in each cycle, her neck muscles contracted, pulling her head to the left with such force that her mattress shook. For nine hours, my husband and I waited for Miss Millie's pain to ease, pain associated with a large sacral decubitus ulcer, pneumonia, depression, and the sheer exhaustion of breathing that had evolved eighteen months after suffering a stroke—cerebrovascular accident. At eighty-five years old, Miss Millie, a southern belle born and raised in New Orleans, was my friend, my older sister, my mother-in-law. A veritable icon of southern gentility, Miss Millie spent her last few weeks in a most unusual place, a facility in Louisiana somewhere between acute hospital care and long-term care, a specialty facility catering to patients who required more sophisticated care than traditional custodial nursing home services.

When Miss Millie passed—no one used the word "died," a vulgar word not used in this small southern town separated from New Orleans by Lake Pontchartrain—we knew all the staff, having helped them care for her during her last week. We knew names and position titles, quite unusual in health care facilities. Everyone wore name tags with large lettering indicating their positions—RN (registered nurse), LPN (licensed practical nurse), CNA (certified nursing assistant), respiratory therapist, and physical therapist. Miss Millie had a Do Not Resuscitate (DNR) order on her chart, congruent with her wishes that she not receive cardiopulmonary resuscitation or advanced cardiac life support. Language on a medical chart, however, becomes real at a bedside, as staff and family members often struggle to determine the difference between comfort measures versus life-saving interventions. After we had decided to remove

Miss Millie's continuous positive airway pressure machine, a young registered nurse one early dawn morning returned her to it, saying it was just too hard for her to breathe without it, the machine requiring less ventilatory effort on her part. A seasoned charge nurse, taking this young nurse under her wing, helped her recognize that this breathing treatment was no longer needed and replaced it with a simple nasal cannula with low-flow oxygen. In that Miss Millie could no longer digest the feeding administered through her gastrostomy tube, this tube was eventually clamped; she continued, however, to receive dextrose 5 percent in water intravenously. As the wound care team, including a plastic surgeon, sought to debride her deep sacral bed sore, we asked that they hold their care, given that such treatment would only escalate Miss Millie's pain unnecessarily. Her chest was noisy, as pneumonia took progressive hold of her lungs, rapidly diminishing the oxygen available to her tissues. She developed seizures. Suctioning her lungs only made the situation worse, removing oxygen as well as mucous.

As her oxygen saturation fell, *the light*, as my husband said, *left her eyes*. The Cheyne-Stokes breathing pattern commenced. *What do you want to do*, the staff asked, including her primary care physician. For comfort, they advised, we could increase her morphine sulfate intravenous pain infusion; as well, an anxiolytic indicated for seizure control—Ativan—could be given intravenously. Both were administered. Comfortably switching from acute care to hospice care, the staff incorporated us invisibly as team members, allowing my husband to carry out Miss Millie's wishes without fear of abandonment, disdainful glances, or disagreeable conversations. Although her last hours were fraught with exhaustive breathing, she had been allowed dignity and respect for her wishes, with her son at her side. In this community specialty facility in a small southern town far from the madding crowd of academic health science centers, Miss Millie's life cycle looped around, her ashes to be scattered across Lake Pontchartrain, a central symbol of her deeply southern life.

Throughout our week with Miss Millie, I watched a health care system operate seemingly effortlessly, with providers secure in their roles, confident in their practice, and at ease in working as teams. A suburban community setting, not an urban university setting: devoid of health professions' students roaming in hallways, eager but tense; absence of the atmosphere of paternalistic control common in health science university care settings. Miss Millie's primary care physician, Greg, visited her each evening, hugging me, and shaking my husband's hand.

Tall, thin, with curly gray-speckled black hair, he leaned against the wall one evening, saying he was tired. It was 7 P.M. He had started his day at 6 A.M.

with rounds of hospital patients followed by forty-eight office visits of patients with either continuing care needs or acute illnesses. He looked forward, he offered, to the end of the summer, when Melissa, a recent nurse practitioner graduate, would join him full time. While she was a graduate student rotating in his practice to learn primary care, Melissa had managed many of his patients as her skills advanced. Smiling, he told us that several patients were annoyed that he would be managing their care until Miss Melissa came on board full-time, once she had passed her board certification as a nurse practitioner. *She will care for the patients down one hall, and I'll care for those on the other side, then we will meet up and compare notes*, said Greg. *We will be a team!* He saw the MD-NP team as a natural one, with improved patient outcomes possible through the relationship. *I am an old-fashioned doctor, I like to sit back and ask my patients how they are doing.* Despite his office manager's desire for him to see as many patients as physically possible every day, he wanted to slow down; maybe see thirty patients instead of forty-eight? Between Melissa and him, perhaps fifty patients could be seen daily, and they could manage hospital and long-term care patients together. Like providers in the North, they were juggling, always juggling the number of patients that must be seen to make ends meet financially. With an overall increase in patients, with a nurse practitioner in his practice Greg could increase revenue cost-effectively. *I don't understand*, he said, *why other doctors don't want to use nurse practitioners more.*

In addition to Greg, we also worked with Randi, a certified respiratory therapist. He explained the positive airway pressure machine to us, indicating early on that he would begin to wean Miss Millie from the machine and let her breathe on her own, thus preventing her from becoming dependent on the device. He was confident in his scope of practice and simply informed the physician of his weaning plan, knowing that Miss Millie was a DNR patient. Leaving her on the device might prolong her life, provided that she could still inhale deeply enough to draw oxygen into her lungs. The device's oxygen-rich flow would prevent tissue deprivation. Leaving her on it indefinitely, however, might also prolong her suffering. He spoke calmly and quietly with us, ensuring that final decisions were ours. He provided information for rational decision making, neither withholding potential negative effects nor overly selling positive effects. His approach was ideal in obtaining informed consent, the process used by a provider to secure consent from a patient—or designated family member—to proceed with a treatment, surgery, or procedure. As he removed the face mask connected to the device, Miss Millie's eyes opened and she blinked that she felt better without the full face mask straps circling her head. Slowly, her breathing became more shallow and rapid, as the very act of inhaling became too difficult. Randi and his teammates were aware that this would happen, and we worked with the team to carefully reposition her for optimum breathing and to medicate her for pain.

We can increase her morphine drip, said the charge nurse, *as a comfort measure*. She carefully and slowly noted that by doing so, her breathing may become depressed; respiratory depression is a negative side effect of morphine. We read worlds into that statement. Her tone, gestures, and facial expression allowed us to increase the morphine drip rate. With each seizure, she also received Ativan. Decisions were left to my husband, with full information and support accompanying each one. The staff moved fluidly between management of chronically ill geriatric patients with acute problems to hospice care, without hesitation or lack of confidence. There were no heroics from providers; the focus remained exclusively on Miss Millie. Hers was a respectful death, shepherded by a confident, secure team.

While in Louisiana, I had remained vigilant, watching the system deliver care, comparing these experiences with my own experiences elsewhere. As is common throughout the country, the acute care delivered at the end of life even surpasses the nature and intensity of care provided in long-term care environments. The battalion includes plastic surgeons and wound teams to manage bed sores; respiratory therapists for breathing-assistive devices; pain management nurses and infectious disease teams to manage pneumonia and infected bed sores; and regimens to turn patients every two hours by nursing staff members. The need for such care is generated by the many consequences of prolonged bed rest in long-term care facilities. Too much care, expensive care, too late. Perhaps, as I mentioned to Miss Millie's physician Greg, nursing homes would benefit from the services of an on-site geriatric nurse practitioner to monitor for these hazards and to initiate treatment prior to the development of complications requiring hospitalization. He and his nurse practitioner Melissa practice prevention in the nursing home, but most doctors still do not want nurse practitioners. Nurse practitioners, Greg believed, would monitor lung sounds, treating early stages of pneumonia before acute respiratory failure developed; review urine samples to note presence of urinary tract infection, treating it early; assess skin, particularly the sacral area, for beginning signs of bedsores, and work with nursing staff to initiate an aggressive turning schedule. Greg and I both knew that the system is skewed to the right—focused on acute illness care, even in a captured nursing home population—and requiring expensive hospitalization rather than preventive geriatric care progressing to hospice care. Righting this system will require the removal of barriers that prevent registered nurses and nurse practitioners to gain full practice, even if

removal is discomforting. And, an entirely different orientation is needed—
health care versus illness care.

Reports by Big Brother

On a breathtakingly cold day in February 2010, with a large black garbage bag
in one hand and wearing a disposable glove on the other, I walked around
the front lawn and sidewalks of the Temple Health Connection building on
West Berks Street, on the perimeter of Temple University's main campus, pick-
ing up trash as the wind tossed it around. The nurse-managed health center,
owned by the Public Health Management Corporation (PHMC) and sponsored
by Temple's Department of Nursing, had been chosen for an on-site review by
the Institute of Medicine/Robert Wood Johnson Foundation Committee (IOM/
RWJF), a committee constituted to explore the future of nursing in the United
States. It was an important day. This prestigious eighteen-member multidisciplinary committee, chaired by Donna Shalala, a political scientist, and co-
chaired by Linda Burnes Bolton, a nurse with a doctorate in public health, had
been charged to assess and transform the nursing profession to ensure affordable, patient-centered, evidence-based quality care. A major focus of the committee was the exploration of issues surrounding nurse practitioner practice:
Did barriers to their practice exist? What was the nature of barriers? How could
barriers be overcome? Deemed an honor to be visited by a sub-group of this
committee, Nancy Rothman galvanized the staff for action on that cold day. We
cleaned, cleared, washed, and repaired anything unsightly. As the sun came
up, we were ready.

As committee members were assisted off a minivan and guided to our
meeting room adjacent to the health center—a large general community activities room used primarily by children—excitement and anticipation thickened.
Nancy had lined up her teammates well in advance, including her community
advisory leaders, clinical staff, students, a collaborating physician, members of
the Public Health Management Corporation, and faculty. While all players may
not have been entirely clear about the reason for this visit, all were absolutely
sure of one thing—Nancy had requested our presence. Nancy is a leader in the
nurse-managed health center movement in Philadelphia, and, through her work
at the National Nursing Centers Consortium and as a member of the National
Committee for Quality Assurance, she provides national nursing leadership.

Located in a Housing and Urban Development (HUD) apartment converted
to serve as a primary care center, the Health Center overflowed with small areas
serving as examination spaces, corners and closets packed with recurring clinical supplies, papers, forms, equipment, pharmaceutical closets, and, in one

room, a small corner desk for a social worker. Crowded, noisy, tight, but work-able, the health center reflected the texture and vibrancy of the very community it served. Enjoying the support and admiration of local residents who received their care at the Health Connection, the center was central to those who lived and worked in this neighborhood. Residents frequently held jobs in health pro-motion efforts funded by federal, state, or local foundation grants and contracts. As Temple employees, they were eligible for tuition remission benefits, thus opening possibilities for advancing their education. A steady-state, win-win situation: operated by PHMC as a federally qualified health center and consis-tent with Temple University's mission, the Health Connection is a prototype of cost-effective, accessible ambulatory primary care. A good choice to visit.

After introductions, those seated in the large circle responded to ques-tions and comments by the committee members present. What types of care are delivered at the center? Who are the providers? How do the nurse prac-titioners and physician of protocol work together? Are there any barriers to the care delivered? What is the referral network used, and how effective is it? What medical documentation system is used? Are the resources adequate to run the center? How does the community advisory council impact the opera-tion of the center? I spoke to my own ability at the Mary Howard Health Center, a sister center also operated by PHMC, to practice autonomously to my full scope of practice, for the first time in my professional career. Neither requiring permission from a physician to practice nor restricted by hospital protocols to implement independent nursing functions, I found it intoxicatingly reward-ing to work in the center. Mike, our Temple nursing faculty president and a geriatric nurse practitioner, addressed our ability at the centers to engage in full evidence-based practice. Sporting a full gray beard, shocking silver-white hair, and holding his bicycle helmet on his lap, Mike expressed our mandate to transform care delivery at our centers from an exclusive illness management orientation to strategies to assist urban residents to embrace healthy lifestyles—from eating habits, to exercise, to violence prevention, regular immunizations, and more. Leaning forward in his folding chair, pants' cuffs tucked into biker boots, Mike struck me as the metaphor for this transformation. Intense, pas-sionate, hardworking, and exceptionally articulate, Mike could speak sponta-neously in any group, at any time. Donald Parks, our collaborating physician, spoke to regulatory restrictions on the number of nurse practitioners that any one physician could work with at a center. Inferring that such restrictions were arcane and not within the best interests of patient care, Donald advocated for full scope of nurse practitioner practice constrained only by the need to main-tain physician collaboration. The committee members listened, occasionally seeking clarification or expansion of an idea. With Nancy skirting the perimeter, hosting light breakfast fare for all present, the site visit ended quietly, with members returning to their van—and back to the IOM.

On October 5, 2010, the IOM/RWJF announced their report—*The Future of Nursing: Leading Change, Advancing Health.* A century earlier, Abraham Flexner, an educator, published his report on medical education funded by the Carnegie Foundation for the Advancement of Teaching—*Medical Education in the United States and Canada: A Report to the Carnegie Foundation for the Advancement of Teaching.* Flexner's 1910 report, which remains the seminal document establishing the primacy of medical education in America, recommended a reduction in the number of medical schools, a standardized curriculum with strict admissions, and strong regulatory boards of medical examiners. Unleashing capitalism, physicians went to the head of the class. Nurses, according to Abraham Flexner and reported by Emily C. Covert in the *American Journal of Nursing* (November 1917), were to serve as "another arm to the physician." The IOM/RWJF report, much like the Flexner report, cited key messages related to nursing education, practice, and regulation. These messages may seem like a recurring dream to nurses who have heard them before, but now they had teeth, given the Supreme Court's affirmation in June 2012 of Public Law 111–148—the Patient Protection and Affordable Care Act. Critically important is the recommendation that nurses practice to the fullest extent of their education and training, with barriers to practice removed. A parallel recommendation promotes seamless academic progression for nurses across educational levels. Unlike the Flexner report, the IOM/RJWF report falls short on specifics, providing, instead, broad generalities that sweep across the large and diverse landscape that is nursing—across the educational preparation spectrum leading to licensure as a registered nurse. Unable to provide specifics, with continued funding provided by the RWJF, Action Coalitions, will be established in successfully competing states to implement strategies and tactics to realize the committee's various recommendations. Successful strategies are anticipated to be replicable, thus solidifying improvements. The IOM/RWJF messages exist in an economic context that has shifted from Flexner's era of free market capitalism to one in which limits are peaking and new markets evolving.

The IOM/RWJF report is silent on entry into nursing practice, differential licensure based on education, and legislation required to initiate regulatory reform. My historical research, coupled with my experiences regarding advanced practice nursing at the University of Medicine and Dentistry of New Jersey, have taught me one irrefutable fact: nursing advances on the basis of legislation and regulatory reform. Neither education alone nor report language alone forwards nurses' scope of clinical practice in the delivery world. Platitudes, belletristic language, and job perks do not trump salary and reimbursement by health insurers for services rendered. Reimbursement follows licensure and certification. The historic evolution of nursing via the hospitalization of America, beginning in the late nineteenth century, forever melded nursing education—and licensure—to hospital practice, hospital training, medicine, and the monosponic economic practices of hospital administrators. The continued practice of awarding the *same* Registered Nurse license to those who graduate from hospital diploma schools, two-year associate degree programs, and four-year baccalaureate degree bolsters the capitalistic practices of medicine and hospital associations.

It is not surprising to me, therefore, that the 671-page IOM/RWJF report, describing the future of nursing as outlined by a predominately non-nurse panel, has spun off requests for demonstration projects. Nor is it surprising that Action Coalitions will not be funded if non-nurse partnerships are not included in applications; after all, it has been a historic pattern that nurses could not be trusted to envision the future of their profession. As the ink dried on the Flexner report, Josephine Goldmark, an industrial efficiency expert, led a team of physicians, hospital administrators, nurses, and science faculty in 1919, supported by funding from the Rockefeller Foundation, on an exploration of nursing education in the United States. The goal: to recommend educational improvements in nursing. Quite unlike Flexner's report, the Goldmark group, in their 1923 publication *Nursing and Nursing Education in the United States*, recommended licensure of nursing's subsidiary workers—the nursing aide—to be trained alongside nurses in hospitals. Two decades later, Ester Lucille Brown, a director at the Russell Sage Foundation, was asked by the National League for Nursing to explore the future of nursing in the second half of the twentieth century. Brown undertook this study from the viewpoint of what was best for society, not from the viewpoint of what was best for nursing. (A theme common in reports on nurses and nursing: the examination of nursing by non-nurses with an eye toward society's needs; the exploration of nursing's or nurses' needs considered too self-serving to examine.) Essentially, Brown recommended in her 1948 report—*Nursing for the Future: A Report Prepared for the National Nursing Council*—enhanced education for both the registered nurse and the practical nurse, with university education appropriate for the registered nurse.

Published shortly after President Harry Truman's Commission on Higher Education report of 1947, Brown's recommendations were overshadowed by the advent of community college degrees for expanding the nursing workforce. The Truman report—*Higher Education for American Democracy*—consistent with recommendations of both the Goldmark and Brown reports, pointed to enlarging the nursing workforce by shortening the education required and introducing ancillary workers.

As I read the IOM/RWJF *Future of Nursing* report, I could not help but recall the aphorism of George Santayana—that those who cannot remember the past are condemned to repeat it—holds fast. Bright colors, prestigious non-nursing organizations, and the promise of funding—all are present in a hardback document, online in pdf or html format, and collapsed into executive summaries within multiple nursing journals. My future and the future of my students are orchestrated by others, as has been true for the past one hundred years. Feeling as if I have lived each of these one hundred years, this paternalistic publication has given me a new perspective. At sixty-one years old, I am militant. Despite my caution about this report, I do look forward to participating in Pennsylvania's Action Coalition.

Reading this document, I know now that legislation is needed to differentiate scope of practice based on education; and I appreciate that reimbursement for evidence-based interventions implemented by registered nurses operating within a scope of practice dictated in legislation and outlined in regulation is possible. The RN-NP team can effect improved health indices documented by outcomes. Are the IOM and the RWJF willing to require legislation for differential licensure? Are they likely to spearhead legislation that would enable the full scope of nurse practitioner practice, galvanizing legislators to sign onto bills to this end? Unlikely. Those changes must be initiated by nurses, militant nurses; and soon. Militancy acknowledges that there are no externalities. The IOM/RWJF report is replete with recommendations for action. Militants act, as noted by Antonio Gramsci in his *Prison Notebooks*. A militant does not recommend. A militant radicalizes action through collapse of boundaries, by a deliberate and willful call for unified action. Ultimately, politically adept, militant nurses, no longer fearful of retaliation or their own freedom, must secure legislative amendments to nurse practice acts, followed by regulatory change.

Newark City Life

The July morning air was muggy, the type of day when your hair clings to the back of your neck and it seems unlikely that you would ever cool down. My sister, Maureen, her best friend, Susan, and her boyfriend, Denny, and I were driving to the airport the morning after racial riots had erupted in Newark. Termed a predictable insurrection by some and an open rebellion by Governor Richard J.

Hughes, the turmoil in Newark in July 1967 was reported by Russell Sackett in *Life* magazine on July 28, 1967, to have resulted in twenty-five deaths, hundreds of injuries, and untold property damage. Denny needed to take back roads to the airport, given that the main streets—Broad Street, Market Street, and Springfield Avenue—were blocked by police. Knowing Newark as well as we all did, it was easy to find our way. The absolute lack of sound, the deadly quiet in the air, was eerie. While the civil rights act of 1964 legislated equality, the deadly trauma of race riots in Newark demanded it and heralded a new era for the city. The four of us in Denny's car knew that life had changed for us.

Maureen's and Susan's excitement about their imminent trip to Miami, Florida, was palpable. They were eighteen years old. This was their long-awaited vacation after working their first year at Newark's Public Service Electric and Gas (PSE&G) Company after graduating from Queen of Peace High School in North Arlington, New Jersey. In the pre-9/11 era, air travel was romantic. As was the norm at that time, they wore new clothes purchased just for traveling. Maureen sported the popular haircut credited to the late British hairstylist Vidal Sassoon—short, angular, cut on a horizontal plane, with one side cut at ear length. Always worried about the appearance of her fine, light brown hair, she had chosen a cut that required minimal management and would withstand well the consequences of Florida's heat and humidity. Susan, a bit more traditionalist, remained faithful to her short, curly bob. Destination—the classic Saxony Hotel on Miami's beachfront. Built in 1948, it was Miami's first opulent, air-conditioned luxury hotel with large guest rooms and complimentary meals. They had saved their money, eager to step into adulthood, complete with cocktails, taxi rides, and flimsy, feminine beach garments to wear as they nested in lounge chairs on the beach. All in the family had reminded them that they wanted souvenirs; Maureen and Susan brought back coconut patties, a delicacy rewarded with big hugs.

Even then, at seventeen years old, I appreciated the ironies of that day.

Newark was always our city. As a child, my buddy Danny and I had walked carefully on railroad tracks to take shortcuts to get to the city. We ate ice cream, I looked at books. Maureen and Susan, on the rare occasions warranting a celebration, would enjoy their lunch breaks at the Pine Room of Hahne's department store on Broad Street in downtown Newark. The Pine Room was the more formal of Hahne's restaurants on the street level; the less prestigious counter-style Maple Room was located on the lower level. As the magnificence of Newark as New Jersey's anchor city in the north slowly dulled, given the confluence of racial unrest, violence, and poverty, Hahne's department store was unsustainable; the Pine Room, however, remained a viable entity until the store closed in 1987. For the majority of their workdays, Maureen and Susan ate Tunas Light Down to Travel (tuna sandwich with mayonnaise, toasted, to go) at the deli on Park Place. Newark excited me; it was my city. As my sister worked at PSE&G, I became a student at Rutgers Newark. Living at home in Kearny, a Scottish town separated from Newark by the Passaic River, I continued to walk to Newark once I had been accepted into the nursing program. I switched my bookstore from my local favorite on Broad Street to the Rutgers bookstore on Central Avenue. I purchased, and read, my anatomy and physiology textbook during the summer prior to my freshman year. I also explored more of Newark, one year post-insurrection. The Newark Public Library, located on Washington Street just a few blocks away from the Rutgers campus, fascinated me. Built in 1901, it has historically served as a meeting place for organizations; in fact, when the New Jersey State Nurses Association was founded that same year, it frequently held business meetings there. My father, a proud member of the carpenter's union, had worked on several large buildings in Newark, including the expansion project at Newark Airport that opened in the early 1970s. As children, Maureen and I would sometimes tour building sites in Newark as my father pointed out construction progress to us.

I loved Newark. It was a city of jobs, education, opportunity, and hope. As racial tension swept through the city, Newark's path veered from its initial position of prominence, as did other cities. I was not, however, afraid of Newark, or of Camden or North Philadelphia. Vigilant, but not afraid. And, as a college student in the sixties, I felt socially responsible to repair Newark. When I was in my psychiatric mental health rotation at Rutgers, I spent time at Overbrook Hospital in Cedar Groove, New Jersey. Built in 1896 as the Essex County Asylum for the Insane, this facility housed hundreds of patients with psychiatric conditions. As psychiatric patients began mainstreaming into smaller residential community facilities, primarily as a result of improved psychotropic medications and newer behavioral therapies, only the fairly recalcitrant patients remained hospitalized when I was a student. My friend, Lois, and I drove together in her Volkswagen Beetle from Newark to Cedar Groove every Tuesday and Thursday while we were assigned at Overbrook.

I was afraid at Overbrook. Locked wards, large three-inch rings of keys, and staff that seemed oddly similar to the patients. Dank, stone walls. Poor lighting. Inadequate staffing. We were to interview select patients, using a stenographer's pad—our questions and comments in the left column, the patient's responses and comments in the right. My first patient, who believed herself to be a typewriter, would move her fingers rapidly over a keypad in the air in front of her and then sing out "ding!" when she got to the end of a line. My individual sessions with my patient did not significantly improve her mental status; nevertheless, I came to understand a lot. I remember my indignation that my patients seemed terminally dirty, with exceptionally poor dental hygiene. In addition to a campaign to collect personal products, including powder, feminine hygiene products, soaps, shampoos, and toothbrushes, I also visited Essex County's Department of Health, seeking funding for more hygiene products as well as assistance in disbursing them. I recall a quick, kind conversation before I was ushered to the door. Disappointed but undaunted, I brought my donated products to Overbrook and gave them to the female patients on my ward, after the head nurse approved. By the next week, everything had vanished.

In addition to rotating at Overbrook, Lois and I also conducted public health visits in Newark. As public health nursing students, we carried a black public health bag—the classic rectangular bag with a latch lock and twelve-inch handles on both sides—with our essentials: thermometer, blood pressure cuff and stethoscope, Band-Aids, gauze, and more. We visited patients in Newark's high-rise apartments, just at a time when they were becoming viewed as forlorn edifices reminiscent of the mid-twentieth-century attempt at urban renewal. Now living at the New Jersey shore, when I close my eyes I can still smell the acid texture of stale urine in corner stairwells. Sometimes a resident would be curled up asleep there. We traveled in pairs, trained to put our public health bags on the old newspapers we placed on the table to keep the bags clean. Likewise, we usually left our coats or jackets in the car, having been cautioned that insects and roaches could easily nest in our coats if we brought them into the apartments. On one trip to the Scudder Homes on West Kinney Street and Irving Turner Boulevard on a snowy day in winter, Lois's Beetle ran out of gas. Four local teenage boys, playing hooky from school, picked up the Beetle and carried it to the gas station on the corner. We each followed a family during this rotation. The mother in my family had multiple sclerosis, a chronic debilitating neurological disease. A young woman, she had young children, all of whom went to the local public school. Perhaps her biggest worry was that her children would be harmed crossing the busy intersection at her street corner, an intersection without a traffic light. She needed an advocate, someone to help her in her campaign to have a traffic light installed at her corner. She and multiple sclerosis had already come to peace with each other; she knew how to manage constipation, skin breakdown, urinary infections, spasms, fatigue, weakness, and side effects of drugs. What she couldn't do was get names on a petition for her traffic light. I took on this task. After I made many door-to-door conversations and phone calls to neighbors, she was able to present her local assemblyman with her petition.

Significantly, I have only vague memories of my classes at Rutgers, but my memories of clinical experiences in Newark facilities and housing units are vivid. I recall the indignity of urban warehousing. I was not at the demolition of the Scudder Homes in the summer of 1996. I would like to have thrown a brick.

One of the sequels to the Newark insurrection was the *Newark Agreements Reached between Community and Government Regarding New Jersey College of Medicine and Dentistry and Related Matters* signed in April 1968, a landmark document forged by community leaders and elected local and state officials that created the University of Medicine and Dentistry of New Jersey (originally titled the New Jersey College of Medicine and Dentistry) to serve as the city's family physician. As Stanley S. Bergen, president of UMDNJ recalled years later, we agreed to be the family physician to New Jersey's most medically underserved population. Certainly this was a unique role, even among academic health sciences universities that typically integrate patient care as an indirect gain to the primary missions of education and research.

I have poured over the *Newark Agreements* intermittently throughout my professional life, attempting to appreciate the passion of the promises made to residents in the aftermath of the 1967 carnage as tanks rolled down Broad Street and soldiers armed with rifles lined major streets. In the immediate post-Newark Agreements era, Governor William Cahill, promoting the establishment of UMDNJ in Newark, solidified the young institution's role when he mandated in his *Special Message to the Legislature* on May 4, 1970, that the university must carry out its mission in relation to the needs of the total community.

Since 1972, the year I graduated with my bachelor's degree from Rutgers University in Newark, my professional choices have been deeply influenced by events in Newark in 1967, flavored by the civil rights and women's rights movements. As an academic administrator, my mantra has consistently been to improve patient care by preparing competent nurses. Quality education is the vehicle to improved health care delivery. As an academic administrator, I am often discouraged from voicing my mantra at meetings. My perspective is not shared. We are about education, not patient care, men without licenses tell me. Given my lifelong perspective—acquired in 1967 in Newark—I cannot help but smile, even laugh.

As I worked at my UMDNJ desk in 1997, I received a call from Stanley Bergen. He was on speaker phone, with a medical school dean and several medical faculties on the call with him. *Fran,* he said, *would you want to offer health care services at the Saint Columba Neighborhood Club in Newark? The medical school was not interested,* he said; *they had other priorities. It would be an opportunity for nurses and nurse practitioners to provide primary care.* Forever cagy, he had me in a corner. Once the nurse practitioner legislation was passed in New Jersey in 1991, I had sought opportunities for our nurse practitioner faculty and students to demonstrate their impact in primary care delivery. Yes, I would be pleased to work with Saint Columba Neighborhood Club. Saint Columba's, a Hispanic community-based organization located on Pennsylvania Avenue in southern Newark, was associated with a Catholic church and elementary school of the same name. A full-service social and welfare organization devoted to local residents, their primary leader—Sister Mary—was eager to add health services to their array of programs. Tall, tough, resilient, and kind, Sister Mary was interested in prevention. Her school children had poor immunization records, a high incidence of pregnancy, and chronic exposure to violence. Could we help her? Yes, we would help. When I came to the club, Sister Mary would ask a local prostitute to sit on my car as a theft deterrent.

While my goal was to provide primary care to club residents as well as those in the local neighborhood, what we accomplished was something quite different. For our nurse practitioner faculty to practice primary care, I needed to obtain a collaborative practice agreement with either a local community physician or one or more physicians from our medical school in Newark. Our medical school faculty locked down on this issue, with the dean saying that he reigned but did not rule, a code that he would not even attempt to influence the chairs of his departments to work with me. It was my responsibility to entice one or more physicians to serve as our collaborating physician.

I turned to money.

I developed a side agreement that would provide 25 percent of our clinical income to our collaborating physician(s), based on revenue obtained from health payers. Despite months of wrangling deals, I could not even entice anyone with money. We would probably not earn enough money to make this venture worthwhile. In the late 1990s, health insurers were beginning to realize that nurse practitioners were now also primary care providers (PCP), and as such, could have panels of patients. A relatively new phenomenon, the nurse practitioner as PCP was not yet fully endorsed by the many physicians who feared loss of income and control. Calling the shots on health insurance committees, physicians continued to influence decisions on which providers would be credentialed. I struggled to understand and navigate the insurance industry, even hiring a lawyer as staff to guide us. And, without a line item in my school's budget to provide health services at the club, I needed to embed community health services as an integral supplement to our academic programs.

In academic year 1998–1999, we moved our UMDNJ school of nursing in a drastically different direction—toward community and primary health care delivery. Given that the faculty already engaged in practice delivery through our approved Nursing Faculty Practice Plan, we now needed to establish a community service arm to complement our academic programs. In 1999, the faculty unanimously endorsed the Community Health Services Program (CHSP), a service unit based initially at the Saint Columba's Neighborhood Club. This action, congruent with the university's mission to serve as Newark's family physician, unified us, giving us a setting within which to function independently. Mission, vision, goals, and objectives later, we worked for years at the club, serving in a variety of roles, including school nurse, immunization nurse, health educator, and health advocate.

Without either the administrative infrastructure to support a full primary care service—health insurance payments, credentialing as primary care providers, billing and receiving mechanisms, laboratory and diagnostic services—nor the physical environment to be licensed by the New Jersey Department of Health as an ambulatory practice, we flourished by doing what Sister Mary and the residents wanted: primary health care. We contracted with the Department of Health to provide childhood immunizations on-site at the club, greatly improving the immunization rates of children at the school and within the neighborhood. Betty and Marta, the registered nurses recruited to provide nursing services full time at the club, designed our clinical programs in concert with club members. By reshuffling our personnel, I was able to shift lines from faculty to professional staff, thus enabling Betty and Marta to join our ranks. Marta, a Hispanic nurse, and Betty, a Spanish-speaking Jewish nurse, magnificently focused on exactly what residents wanted rather than on providing primary care disease diagnosis and management. Residents could go to a local "doc-in-the-box" or a hospital emergency department for disease care; what they wanted from us was help in becoming healthier. Lifestyle management to control blood pressure; better diets for diabetes management; stress reduction regimens to combat depression; drug management instruction for HIV-positive residents; lower rates of teenage pregnancies and sexually transmitted infections. These were clear, manageable requests that opened new pathways for independent practice for registered nurses.

Even lifestyle management required money, however. With minimal routine funding from the school of nursing, our work at the club was at risk. Phone bills, computers, paper supplies, routine recurrent clinical supplies—from Band-Aids to immunizations—became expensive, threatening to close us if we did not find a sustainable source of funding. I went to a friend at our University Hospital. Our chief executive officer knew that the university would not name our CHSP at the club as a university-designated ambulatory practice, so he provided supplies under the table. On a monthly basis, I gave him a list of needed supplies; he then had them sent to us. We survived, rotating students at the club to expand services.

Betty and Marta, however, were not satisfied with simple survival. They were concerned about the fate of young girls in the neighborhood, particularly given the common desire for early pregnancy as a symbol of adulthood. With grand flare and excitement, Betty announced that they would establish the Baby-Think-It-Over program at the club's health center. Betty, a confident New York baker who had previously owned a flourishing bakery in Queens, announced in her deep, resonant voice that *the program would be great!* With Marta quietly at her side, Betty barreled forward to begin the program, again with start-up funds from reallocation within the School of Nursing. Begun in 1993 by Richard Jurmain, an aerospace engineer in California, the program immersed young children—girls and boys—in parenting, from sleepless nights, to crafting welfare budgets, to visits to the health center for immunizations, and more. Elementary school children, usually sixth graders, would have a baby simulator for two weeks, all the while monitored by Betty and Marta. Called over the elementary-school intercom that it was their turn to have their baby evaluated at the health center, the parents of a baby simulator would go to the center, wait in the waiting room, review their weekly budget with a staff member, and then have their baby examined by Marta—a grueling experience of interrupted childhood, poverty and sleeplessness. Some of the children asked to return the baby simulators; we said *No, this is your child and he is your responsibility.*

Betty and Marta effected change. Pregnancy rates declined. Their program caught the attention of a local legislator—Robert Menendez, a Democrat from Hoboken and U.S. representative in Congress. Representative Menendez visited the health center amid flashing cameras and reporters, a Kodak moment. Promising to help find us sustainable funding for our services within this primarily Hispanic community, Congressman Menendez went on to other things. With our community advisory board, faculty, and staff supporting this initiative, we were undaunted. We turned to the Robert Wood Johnson Foundation (RWJF) for a program grant. In 1998, we received funding for three years. Thrilled and compulsive, I bought a large wall calendar and highlighted dates for deliverables—project reports and data trends. Focusing our efforts on locally identified health needs, our staff, faculty, and community allies emphasized programs for improving health of children and adolescents. As our three-year grant closed, Betty and I were invited to a conference at RWJF at its headquarters on Route 1 North, near Princeton, New Jersey. Their mission—to improve the health and health care of all Americans—evolved from the philosophy of

Robert Wood Johnson, the World War II brigadier general who built Johnson & Johnson into a leading world company. The foundation, an independent philanthropy evolved from Johnson & Johnson, funds programs targeting equality in health care delivery to all Americans.

As we took our seats at a large conference table seating all grant recipients who had recently closed their programs, we were nervous. Having worked for years in local neighborhoods in Newark, I was impressed with the ostensible appearance of wealth. We took turns describing our programs and outcomes. Betty presented our program. Presenter after presenter closed with comments on sustainability. Not all programs would be continued when the grants ended. Sustainability was our responsibility; RWJF provided initial funding only. As program administrators provided their stories, I began to focus on their "next steps"—their efforts to continue programs without grant dollars. Not all programs could apply as federally qualified health centers; we could not, given our university status. The providers at the grand RWJF table were not all versed in sustainability; I gradually became leery of RWJF, wondering if they would at least share in the responsibility to explore the next steps for funding. At my most cynical, I felt that Betty and I would become poster images for RWJF to demonstrate its goodwill to communities. We were tokens to impress the public of the foundation's good work. The smiles, gentility, impressive luncheon, and grand building could easily be exchanged for continued guidance on sustainability. I was not sufficiently grateful. As the Saint Columba Catholic Church began to lose parishioners, its revenue plummeted and eventually the elementary school was closed. With it, the health service closed. While the university supported our efforts conceptually, it would not support us as an ambulatory practice site. We closed along with the school closure.

Refusal to Succeed

I was idealistic and naïve, Carman mused, as he and I reminisced in 2011 about our long-term professional colleagueship that began in 1995 at the University of Medicine and Dentistry of New Jersey (UMDNJ). Carman, the chairman of the Department of Family Medicine in the School of Osteopathic Medicine (SOM) located on the university's Stratford campus, had eagerly joined forces with me to demonstrate that interdisciplinary education was more than a mere aphorism. Without an eyebrow raised in skepticism, Carman's family practice faculty and the School of Nursing's nurse practitioner faculty met in the dean's large conference room in what Davida, our administrative coordinator, called the White House. The White House—SOM's Academic Center opened in 1993 as the school's linchpin for teaching activities—was the pride of the campus, a state-of-the-art center with classrooms, a walking track and gym facilities, spacious library, and a dining area. Carolyn, our assistant dean of nursing on the Stratford campus, was ebullient, laying out our course schedule and curriculum content, hoping to coordinate teaching topics with family medicine's curriculum. What was an insurmountable barrier in Newark was an easy task with SOM in Stratford. Given that both nurse practitioners (NPs) and osteopathic physicians must learn a common core of skills and knowledge related to conducting physical examinations, we quickly found ourselves bartering topics. We'll teach head, eye, ear, neck, and throat, offered an SOM faculty. We'll do the lecture on respiratory, Carolyn offered, noting that we would include allergic rhinitis along with asthma and chronic obstructive pulmonary disease. Our students, first-year SOM and NP students admixed in both the classroom and practice settings, a major step toward meeting the elusive goal of teaching and learning together. Years later, Carolyn referred to this period of our joint history as Camelot, a time when, through force of personalities, we realized our aims. There was, you see, no magic in Camelot. There was only will.

Our will expanded to include interdisciplinary practice as Carolyn forged a relationship with the Reverend Floyd White III, an informal, powerful leader within the Camden community. Diminutive in size and larger than life in persona, the reverend had iconic status. He was the pastor of the small Woodland Avenue Presbyterian Church, located on Eighth Street and Woodland Avenue in Camden, which he framed as the central hub for a faith-based, nonprofit organization created in 1997—the Woodland Community Development Corporation—to provide social services to low-income families in Camden. A soft-spoken, well-dressed, pragmatic believer in social reform, "the Rev," as we called him, operated in the interstices between community-based organizations and local politics. Capable of swaying opinion in board rooms as well as in tenant association meetings, the Rev had an agenda, and the capacity to make it happen. As we walked down Eighth Street, he in the middle with one arm reaching over Carolyn's shoulder and the other over mine—a scene we all recognized was far from Kansas, or Oz—we committed to providing health services at this church. Federal faith-based, social programs began in 1996, when Congress enacted the first Charitable Choice initiative. The appreciation that churches, steadfast pillars of stability in urban centers, could participate in social welfare and health programs awakened politicians, academics, and health providers to a new venue of practice—and funding. Thirty years after the racial insurrection in Newark, Camden's faith community, under the Rev's cagey politics, liberated itself from the sole discretion of standard governmental leadership.

The Rev wanted health services offered in his church, but his operational definition of "service" was wide open, focusing on education and advocacy more than on direct primary care. He asserted that teenagers in his church, for example, needed to learn about HIV transmission and safe sex, in sessions in his church without parents present. He knew his community intimately, as Betty and Marta knew the Saint Columba Neighborhood Club community in Newark. Immunization programs, antiviolence campaigns, lifestyles to prevent hypertension and diabetes, and more: these were the health services he wanted us to implement. Effervescent like an Alka-Seltzer tablet, Carolyn easily won the support of her Stratford faculty to work on faith-based initiatives. The result: the design of a Church Nurse Program, a ten-week program offered in collaboration with several churches in Camden, orchestrated under the Rev's and Carolyn's powerful leadership. After conducting conversations with church members—focus group sessions, which are key in qualitative research and program design—and nursing faculty, Carolyn's team developed a program based on the identified needs of community residents. Church nurses, sometimes called Parish Nurses, run the gamut from being licensed registered nurses to community residents without formal training in health.

In our case, we offered an educational program to women who had informally self-identified as "Church Nurses," helpers dressed completely in white uniforms and white shoes who offered assistance to parishioners overcome during church services. As the Rev said, *being overcome may be due to the power of the Spirit, or possibly due to a stroke.* Church Nurses, whether licensed or untrained, needed to know the difference. Our program included ten evening sessions, each with two parts. First, with the help of a small grant, we offered dinner; then we taught a topic, often with demonstrations and return demonstrations. Food, it turned out, was a valuable incentive; in fact, a focal point for each session. Warm, boisterous social events, these training sessions were successful. Church Nurses attended. Sessions included influenza vaccines (why, when, and where to get them), how to take a pulse, signs of a stroke, HIV transmission, sexually transmitted infections (and how to prevent them), baby care, lifestyle changes to manage diabetes and hypertension, and social and welfare services. Here was a banquet of externalities. Carolyn graduated several classes of church nurses, with the Rev beaming at her side.

With the Church Nurse Program a success, the Rev encouraged our increased involvement in the Camden community. He introduced Carolyn and me to Arnold Byrd, executive director of the Camden County Council on Economic Opportunity (CCCOEO). Arnold, a shy, gruff man with a tough appearance, had run the CCCOEO for almost a lifetime. A private, nonprofit agency offering social welfare services to Camden's low-income families since 1965, CCCOEO was housed in a magnificent former city library building on the corner of Broadway and Royden Street. Brusque and short on words, Arnold endorsed the idea of a health services component to the CCCOEO; it was the only program missing from his panoply of services. He gave us two rooms at the extreme end of the central corridor, both approximately fourteen by sixteen feet in dimension. Thrilled, we outfitted the rooms as an ambulatory practice. We washed, vacuumed, cleaned, and converted one room into an examination room; the second room served as our office—complete with file cabinet for patient records and other office equipment. Here was our primary care facility, a complementary delivery component to the health education and advocacy services offered at Woodland Church and through the Church Nurses Program.

Carolyn invited her nurse practitioner faculty to provide primary care at our newly designated Camden Community Health Center. Converting a faculty line into a fund for faculty practice, Carolyn enticed faculty to practice at the center, providing services supplemental to those provided by patients' primary care providers. To provide such service within the regulatory parameters of the New Jersey State Board of Nursing, we turned to Carman, our colleague in the School of Osteopathic Medicine. As with our interdisciplinary education efforts, Carman again signed on as our collaborating physician without hesitation. In fact, he signed on his department as well, so that we could have alternate physicians as needed. *Had you been at all reticent to serve as our collaborating physician?* I asked years later. *No*, he said with his charming, quick smile. *Nurse practitioners are on the front line, just like us. They don't extend medical care, they improve it*, he stated. *They are also primarily female, and we need more female primary care providers.* A major advantage of nurse practitioners, he thought, is that they are lifelong learners; they embrace what they don't know and then learn about it. Surprisingly, Carman also said what I had thought to be true for many years—like osteopaths, nurse practitioners are underdogs; they have to prove their worth all the time. In our world resplendent with the arrogance of allopathic physicians—MDs—both osteopaths (Doctors of Osteopathy, DOs) and NPs are natural partners, neither needing to impress or control the other. Our relationship, according to Carman, was stronger than the requirements outlined in the regulations. Rather than having a specific process of reviewing medical records written by NPs, we had instead a true collaboration: we just called each other whenever we needed to, with Carman triaging our center's patients to specialists within SOM and helping them to obtain health insurance. Carman eventually expanded our Camden

Center services by providing pediatric care on site each Saturday morning, with an attending physician and students offering care.

By 2010, the UMDNJ School of Nursing had withdrawn from the Camden Community Health Center. SOM, however, remained onsite, providing what they termed the Saturday Clinic. I was saddened when I learned in spring of 2011 that nursing had withdrawn from the center. Carman said that nursing had stated that the center did not conform to state regulations as an ambulatory practice site; thus, they withdrew. Without need for language, Carman and I understood the code. Sustaining a community service mission requires dedication and passion, a willingness to appreciate the return on investment through indirect gains to the academic mission. Such a call to service takes time, money, and risk taking. There is nothing simple about managing urban residents with complex comorbid illnesses. It's easier to close up shop than assume risk.

Failure to Thrive

I had dealt with non-risk-taking behavior earlier in my career at UMDNJ. Concurrent with the Camden programs with the Reverend Floyd White, Arnold Byrd, and Carman, I had sought community partnerships with groups in Newark in addition to the Saint Columba Neighborhood Club. The intent: to move curricula into the neighborhoods of Newark for two reasons—first, congruence with the mandates of the Newark Agreements; and second, to enhance the relevancy and marketability of our curricula. When the UMDNJ chapter of the American Association of University Professors (AAUP) acknowledged the value of our offer to full-time faculty to matriculate into our post-master's nurse practitioner program, one faculty from our joint associate degree program with Middlesex County College enrolled in the Adult Health track. She paid severely for doing so. Faculty generally were averse to the program, believing that once completed, they would be assigned to working at community health sites, delivering primary care. They erected a wall that any potentially willing faculty member would have to be very agile, confident, and self-assured to leap over. Lina was a quiet woman who became accustomed to being alone within her own faculty group, seeking instead validation from me and others on the Newark campus. Once graduated, Lina expressed a willingness to work at a community site in Newark. Adjacent to the UMDNJ Newark campus were two housing projects, one the Georgia King Village and the other the New Hope Village. I went to both, with the strength of the university's commitment to the Newark community as my defense.

Georgia King Village, located on the corner of Bergen Street and Cabinet Street, opposite the Stanley S. Bergen Building—the former Martland Hospital, the city hospital for Newark—housing UMDNJ administrative offices as well as the Schools of Nursing and Health Related Professions, has 422 low-cost Housing and Urban Development (HUD) housing units owned in 2011 by a Florida firm. In conversations with their tenants' association, it was understood that this community wanted services for their children, from well-child to acute illness care. Episodic illness care demanded collaboration with faculty in our New Jersey Medical School (NJMS). NJMS, the oldest of the university's academic units, was fortunate have to several well-known faculty, including one endowed professor, an expert in HIV/AIDS care. With a community affairs colleague at my side, I met with a pediatric medical administrator in a conference room at Georgia King Village on a warm summer's day, looking forward to touring him around the facility that we had been given as a health center. The meeting was surprisingly short. Once I invited my medical colleague to consider serving as our collaborating physician, he cut to the bottom line: *yes, I will do it if I get half of any money you collect.* My community affairs colleague stood up and began pacing. I agreed to pay 25 percent of any revenue we received, knowing well that we had not yet been credentialed by any health insurance company. He said he would consider the offer, and then left the village without seeing the health site. This venture became increasingly complex, with my medical colleague not only ultimately refusing to serve as our collaborating physician, but additionally, in the presence of a senior university administrator, promising that he would stop nurse practitioner gains in the state, working through the New Jersey Board of Medical Examiners. Although nurse practitioners continued to function despite his threat, we shut down our Georgia King Village efforts, informing the community that we simply did not have the resources at that time to do a good job. Greed and the distasteful use of power soured my desire to offer services at the Village, despite the community's request. What was possible in Stratford and Camden with osteopaths was not possible in Newark with allopaths. What was possible with osteopaths was not consistently possible with nursing faculty, many of whom during this time were unsupportive of nurse practitioners.

We did, however, offer services at New Hope Village, a Section 8 HUD housing community with 122 apartments located on West Market Street, two blocks away from the UMDNJ campus. The tenants' association president welcomed us, inviting us to use both a small first-floor room for examinations and a larger community room for health education programs. Lina was embraced by this community. An adult nurse practitioner, Lina was a serious, dedicated, and extraordinarily dependable clinician at New Hope. Because we could not offer primary care services without an agreement with a collaborating physician, we ultimately did more. Lina proved to be passionate about primary health care, with a focus on health education and advocacy. The New Hope Village Health Center (the Center), within just a few months, began offering services Monday through Friday with four hours on Saturdays. By reshuffling personnel on our Newark campus, I was able to have three nurse practitioners share one staff line and thus offer services daily, with evening hours offered three days per week. On a website created in 1997 and remaining live in 2012, one young resident noted in 1997 that *the nurse practitioners take care of us. They teach us how to take care of our health, how to improve our health, and they help us when we need special care.* The nurses ran workshops on special health issues and invited other health care providers to visit for special health needs. Based on residents' expressed needs, children at NHV were offered computer classes aimed at exposing them, in the mid- to late 1990s, to the internet. The New Hope Kids on the Net program eventually expanded, allowing children to increase their computer skills under the guidance of the university's Academic Computing Services experts.

Despite these complexities, results nonetheless occurred. The UMDNJ nursing faculty who provided health education and advocacy, as well as primary and secondary prevention services, were given teacher contact equivalencies (TCEs), important units of faculty productivity measurement outlined in our teachers' contract. Faculty practice is commonplace within academic health science universities. The provision of patient services by licensed registered nurse or nurse practitioner faculty has long been my mantra. Maintaining competence is a minimal expectation for licensed faculty.

What has been interesting in my administrative experience at Temple—a comprehensive public research university—is the institutional culture regarding payment for clinical services provided by faculty. If faculty members receive their salary for contact hours with students and equivalent clinical services with patients, then is it really double-dipping to provide them with a clinical supplement? My response: No. Faculty salaries are not comparable to clinical salaries; academic salaries are lower, attracting faculty with promises of lifestyle satisfaction and the time to engage in scholarship and research. Often, these indirect incentives may actually attract those who no longer wish to practice, resulting in disengagement from the very clinical knowledge and skills they are expected to teach their students. And, although Pennsylvania—like other states—allows state employees to hold outside employment up to 20 percent of their time in the state position, this method of practice does not ensure that students will have the luxury of being mentored by faculty as they engage in their practice site. *You can't have an incentivizing faculty practice plan. Temple won't approve double-dipping,* says a finance officer. My medical school colleagues, however, have a spontaneous reply: Of course you need to incentivize clinical faculty, both to retain them and to get their salaries competitive with practice salaries. While nurse practitioners are reimbursable as primary care providers, our practice plan is dormant. We fail to thrive. We falter at growth and development milestones, become irritable, easily distracted, and perform poorly in learning situations. Failure to thrive—or, institutional refusal to allow success—is an insurmountable barrier to progress.

Disruptive Concepts

From the fourteenth floor window of the office of UMDNJ's senior vice president for administration and finance, one could see Newark twinkling in the early evening glow of street lights and building reflections, a romantic scene played against a deep cobalt-blue backdrop, with New York City's Twin Towers and Empire State Building framing the landscape. In 1999, administrators at UMDNJ faced an odd dilemma. Treatment regimens for patients infected with the Human Immunodeficiency Virus (HIV) were succeeding; patients were living longer, fending off opportunistic infections, with progression to Auto-immune Deficiency Syndrome (AIDS) no longer an inevitable consequence. In 1996, UMDNJ, along with several colleague institutions in Newark, established Broadway House for Continuing Care. Broadway House was build under assumptions generated by the knowledge of HIV and AIDS obtained in the late 1980s and early 1990s. Essentially a hospice for terminally ill HIV/AIDS patients, Broadway House operates under state regulations as a long-term care facility. Highly active antiretroviral therapy (HAART) advanced more than medical care for HIV/AIDS patients; additionally, it transitioned Broadway House from a hospice environment to a long-term care facility with young patients, the majority of whom were ambulatory. Neither terminally ill nor well enough to return to community living, these residents lived at Broadway House, their previous lifestyle behaviors and psychological complexities unmasked by their antiretroviral therapies.

Broadway House, said Jim, the senior vice president, *might close.* It was becoming a problem to manage. The residents were no longer confined to bed, with nurses' expertise in acute care providing complex management regimens that prolonged life until opportunistic infections overwhelmed their immune capacity, resulting in death. Residents were now young, ambulatory, with substance abuse histories and psychiatric management needs incongruent with the expertise of the professional staff. HAART disrupted Broadway House rapidly, as if a cyclone had overturned it, exposing behavioral problems mandating a radically different clinical skill set. A decision had to be made to keep it open, to close it, or to expand it. Jim and Stanley Bergen, the president emeritus of UMDNJ—on whose watch Broadway House had been established—needed to make a decision, but they wanted confirmation of the problems existing at Broadway House in this postcyclone era. They gave me an internal grant to study the facility, to tease out the issues and to make recommendations to them in six months.

I gathered a team. Colleagues at our partner institution, the New Jersey Institute of Technology, joined nursing faculty and graduate students at UMDNJ to concretely plan our study. An economist, in collaboration with other faculty, explored the financial structure of Broadway House, interviewing financial officers and delving into state regulations for long-term care as well as Medicaid reimbursement to the facility. A second team, including graduate nursing students, outlined a qualitative and quantitative research approach to address the complex context of the place. A few of us spent time on every shift at Broadway House, enjoying time with patients at night, those who couldn't sleep and ate bagels with us in the magnificent central hallway of the facility. Broadway House was established in the former Essex Catholic High School building on Broadway in Newark. The building—listed in the National Register of Historic Places—was built in 1915 as the headquarters of the Mutual Benefit Life Insurance Corporation, a company chartered in 1845 and dissolved in 2001. It was sold to the archdiocese of Newark in 1979, becoming the Essex Catholic High School. When the population of HIV/AIDS patients began to overwhelm the capacity of acute care hospitals in Newark in the mid-1990s, Broadway House was established in this magnificent building with vaulted, elaborately painted ceilings, marble flooring, and large rooms redesigned for long-term-care resident housing. On benches in the central hall of this building, we chatted with residents using our standing interview schedule, enriched by their sheer willingness to discuss their diagnoses and stresses. We learned that most residents relied on God's mercy and their mothers' love. We also studied patterns of nursing care delivery, using instruments designed for this purpose. Staff, like residents, easily expressed their concerns. Patients who have passes, seek and obtain drugs. Prostitutes prowled the facility, as did drug dealers. Most patients, staff said, were sexually active. They worried about residents' use of condoms; were residents spreading the virus?

As requested, we provided our recommendations within six months. It had been an intense immersion experience in HIV/AIDS care, quite unlike any of our past experiences in research. The facility, we believed, mandated a shift from an acute medical care perspective to a subacute, community-oriented psychiatric/mental health orientation. More, rather than fewer, beds were needed. Likewise, nurse practitioners in psychiatric/mental health were needed to complement the medical care provided by the full-time adult nurse practitioner and part-time physicians. I met with Jim in fall 2000, asking him to review the draft report; I would subsequently give him the revised, final document. *You academics*, he laughed, *we don't have time for re-drafts!* The report was transmitted, in real time, to the state's Commissioner of Health and Senior Services. In December 2000, our team made a presentation to the commissioner in her Trenton office. Broadway House made the shift. It hired a psychiatric nurse practitioner, blending physical care within a broader context acknowledging the psychosocial demands of this unique population of residents. It also received increased state funding, additional beds, and a new administrative team—including both the president/chief executive officer and the executive director, a registered nurse.

Over a decade later, I hold this experience as one of the most meaningful in my life. In light of the consequences of a disruptive therapy—HAART—a leader, Stanley Bergen, faced the situation head-on, willing to interrupt the status quo, accepting the possible outcome of closure of the very facility he had created. Here was a leadership trait to tuck away for future use, as needed.

More of the Same

Leaders of Independence Blue Cross (IBC), in a meeting with deans and directors of nursing education programs in Philadelphia in 2011, sought advice regarding new investments in nursing that would positively impact the profession. What should their foundation invest in to reap the most benefit? After years of scholarship support for nursing students, they now sought new ideas, new venues to fund nursing generally and, thus, to improve patient outcomes. In a large conference room on the forty-fourth floor, approximately twenty nursing education deans and directors met with the social mission executives of the organization. In this long rectangular room, with a majestic view overlooking Philadelphia, we offered alternatives for future investments. In my years at Temple, I had come to appreciate that the deans of Drexel University, Villanova University, the University of Pennsylvania, and Thomas Jefferson University established the tone and directions for nursing in the city. While not all were present at this IBC meeting, those present managed to control the conversation, with an interesting assumption of righteous authority. They called for fellowships for nurse faculty in the area of health policy. With teleological certainty, those present at the table nodded heads affirmatively, although I found it a boring funding alternative.

When the conversation drifted to the financial support of nurses as they academically progressed from associate degrees to more advanced nursing degrees, I became interested. Nursing has enjoyed the financial support of the federal government—the Nurse Training Act—and employer tuition reimbursement for decades, often, I have thought, generating a unique ethos. Nurses sometimes say they cannot advance in their education unless they are funded. While other professions have not had the generous financial support as nursing has, their members do manage somehow to obtain graduate education. Those who wish to advance, do so, seeking funding as needed. When I suggested that perhaps nurses have an entitlement mentality with regards to their continued education, the assumed nurse leaders present crushed my suggestion. The atmosphere was tense; I pushed on, noting that we might capitalize on the language of disruptive technology to destroy nursing's metaphor of a nursing education ladder. The ladder concept frames language of accelerating nursing programs, providing advanced standing in programs based on past education and experience. When I suggested burning the ladder and acknowledging that higher education in nursing needed to be legitimized in regulation and licensure, with different scopes of practice based on education, the tension dissipated into laughter. *That will never happen*, proclaimed the self-identified leaders present. *Look at North Dakota—they tried differential licensure based on education and they failed. So what?* I claimed, *politics and power aside, it must happen if nursing is to advance as a profession.* Why else undertake baccalaureate education if graduates are licensed to perform the same as associate degree and hospital diploma graduates? When I suggested that we were deceiving ourselves and the public, it was, thankfully, at the end of our allotted hour. The next day I received an e-mail from an IBC representative, seeking my response to a Survey Monkey questionnaire regarding the proposal for nursing fellowships to be sponsored by the organization's newly established foundation. That was that.

That same month, trying a different tactic, I visited a foundation that had provided significant funding to nursing programs. I sought permission to utilize some of those funds for an alternate purpose: to fund graduate students' evidence-based clinical doctoral projects in their final year of study. While disappointed in the rejection of my proposal, what was distressing but more interesting was the conversation that followed the rejection. Resoundingly rejecting the need for a clinical doctoral degree for nurse practitioners, the foundation executive and I engaged in a conversation about the time it took to get a degree in nursing. She supported the need to accelerate nursing programs, to graduate nurses efficaciously, to get them into the workplace generating income as soon as possible. I countered with a different hegemony, advocating for deceleration, for the need to integrate the knowledge and skills of research into the practice of primary care in a less frenetic, fast-paced curriculum graduating our students one or two semesters before those of other disciplines graduate theirs. Education in nursing is critical, just as it is for other disciplines, I posited. My colleague's beliefs in providing a workforce quickly and in accelerating students in curricula linked to a tight educational-ladder approach without benefit of time to get a degree silenced my language of nursing's nascent entry into primary care, mandating evidence-based practice.

That evening I explored online images of burning ladders, weighing the possibility of creating personal nursing education stationary with this image as a logo. Or perhaps the image of a person with her head in the sand? Either image might imply the skullduggery of a field insisting on retaining the myth of a nurse is a nurse is a nurse, irrespective of education. The anti-education foundation of nursing pervades its ethos, solidifying its lowly place in the delivery system. Nurse practitioners could not enjoy the pursuit of evidence-based practice research. Why? Because it might take more time! I kept clicking ladder images.

The Devil You Know

Follow the money. This is a hoary adage that commonly guides the work of university development officials. With over three decades of experience in higher education, I have found following money to be a core capitalistic guiding principle, irrespective of stated institutional mission, vision, or goals. As public support for higher education dwindles, university development teams look to support initiatives for new funding. In a tenure-driven system, individual faculty vies for first base; in the grant world, this translates to being the principal investigator on grants. It is difficult to form teams in a situation in which everyone wants to be the first among equals. In my role as dean of nursing at UMDNJ, I found myself in rooms with colleagues who were encouraged to join forces with other schools to mount efforts, for example, to educate at-risk populations about HIV/AIDS management regimens, or efforts to reduce sexually transmitted infections. It is difficult, however, to herd cats. Faculty sometimes coalesce around an initiative, if there is funding in it for them, their department, or their school. The sheer capaciousness of the competitive spirit among faculty, however, can doom collaborative projects, despite the allure of cash.

On a sunny day in Philadelphia in August 2011, several people convened in the waiting area outside Temple University's Advancement Office, located in Sullivan Hall. Erected in 1935 as PWA Project #1326, Sullivan Hall was dedicated as Temple's library in a ceremony attended by President Franklin Delano Roosevelt. Upon passing through the historic wooden doors with their large, ornate iron handles, you walk up a short staircase of grooved stone stairs to enter a large atrium. The Advancement Office, located on the main level, is framed richly in glass, with a spacious and welcoming waiting area. Wealth lives here. It is a very impressive office, as is the building. Named after Thomas D. Sullivan, founder and president of the Terminal Warehouse Company, who donated $278,000 to the construction of the building, the library was completed with PWA funds—$550,000—in 1936. Somewhat cramped in a small conference room to begin explorations on community service projects supported by Temple schools, those invited—from nursing, social work, podiatry, dentistry, medicine, and pharmacy—described their work in communities in Philadelphia. Within short order, the group jockeyed to advocate their views of how health services delivery could be improved in North Philadelphia. Medical-centered health delivery system? Patient-centered delivery system? Perhaps an integrated team approach to health care delivery with the patient at the center? The meeting concluded as everyone finished lunch, the Advancement officer indicating that minutes would be mailed to everyone soon. Handshakes, nods, a sense of satisfaction that the meeting had been a success. I felt otherwise.

Despite my recurrent sense of hopeless déjà vu, I admit having been encouraged by the enthusiasm and language of one member at that conference table—the dentist. We are not dealing with minority health in North Philadelphia, but rather, he said, the majority's health, since the population was predominantly labeled as minorities. He spoke urgently of community involvement in any effort we planned. His passion, combined with his humor, intrigued me. Shortly after this, a pediatric medical faculty member who served as our collaborating physician for a school-based health initiative invited me to meet with an internal medicine faculty member to explore opportunities for nurse practitioner students. A team was forming—the nurse, pediatrician, internal medicine physician, and dentist. We began meeting, sharing each other's views about Temple's future in health care, like-minded in our belief that change was possible, primarily due to new leadership on the campus. Our newly recruited leader did not require instruction on the role of nurse practitioners, nor did he disagree that baccalaureate-prepared registered nurses were grossly underutilized in primary care. As we continued our planning—our goal being the establishment of a horizontally integrated, patient-centered health home provided in partnership with a partner capable of obtaining the critical important designation as a federally qualified health center—others joined. Soon, for our first meeting, we needed name tags for all present, including some from the university's Advancement Office and Office of Government and Public Affairs.

As I prepared for this first meeting, I began to feel a familiar sense of pride, one that becomes increasingly rare with age. Under new leadership, clinicians were encouraged to take ownership of primary care for the host local community. With a shared vision and a common language, I dared to hope for change. If a multidisciplinary patient-centered program emerged, perhaps there could be expansion of our primary health care initiative within my department.

In the past, I had lived with risk and thrived. In the present, I longed for more of that.

It is good, I learned yet again, to be cautious of hope and pride.

A major grant was submitted for a patient-centered initiative, but nurse practitioners were not named as primary care providers. Ultimately not funded, this grant was critiqued as not being innovative in the face of the country's health needs. Nursing's failure to thrive has historically had multiple sources of origin, not the least of which was the dogged refusal to recognize the roles of registered nurses and nurse practitioners as outlined by regulations and law. Contentedly trapped in old worldviews, the bullies—what else shall we call them?—were afraid of change. And, in an interdisciplinary education initiative, we had again been elbowed to the edge by scheduling, a familiar tactic that seems innocuous but rests at the heart of most matters in health care delivery. Interdisciplinary programming was planned for summer months, a time when neither our students nor faculty were available. There was no way forward. I had to withdraw nursing's participation in what had been transformed primarily into a medical school interdisciplinary initiative.

The inevitable e-mail exchange followed.

He said: *I am disappointed at your action.*

She said: *I, too, am disappointed.*

That was the end of it. Nearing the end of my career, I now appreciate that to lead is to be less fearful of disruption. For in nursing, leadership—to lead truly and firmly, not simply to manage—is a disruptive concept.

Epilogue

Within the particular context of nursing practice, to lead is to be disruptive. The act of leading disrupts a status quo, invigorating context, welcoming change. When enacted by a marginalized group, leading disrupts. This relationship between leading and disrupting is not linear, but rather pan-dimensional and perhaps best symbolized by the mathematical operator: ↔. The symbol, however, is context specific.

Memoirs, and the narratives contained in them, are like that as well. Ben Yagoda, who has written a fine book about the history of the memoir, tells his readers that the genre is to be understood as a factual account of the author's life. But there is a qualification: a certain leeway with the facts is expected. Why? Because writers, Yagoda tells us, have all kinds of agendas, from score settling to political action.

Aside from a change of name to protect the innocent, what you have read in these pages is factual. The qualifier, "as far as I can tell," is implicit in any statement of a fact because the act of telling involves language, as slippery a tool as any invented by humans. Facts exist; our rendering of them, however, involves interpretation. Here is a fact from the last line of the memoir you have last read: "For in nursing, leadership—to lead truly and firmly, not simply to manage—is a disruptive concept." The need for disruption is, I propose, a fact. How is that fact to be interpreted in the context of health care delivery in 2012?

Economically, as David Harvey has demonstrated in *The Enigma of Capital and the Crises of Capitalism* (2010), economic expansion of 3 percent of America's compound rate of growth is deemed healthy. For our patient to remain well on such a high-caloric diet, however, is unlikely. As Harvey demonstrates, the 2008 financial collapse is evidence of the environmental, market, profitability, and special constraints facing the current capitalist model of growth in America. His metaphor of health is used consistently. Can capitalism survive the present trauma? he asks. Yes, he affirms, but at what cost? Surrender of rights and assets, from housing to pension rights, environmental degradation, and reduction in living standards are the costs of continuing to adhere to a 3 percent pattern of growth of the gross domestic product.

Within this framework, liberation of women becomes central to a way forward. The feminization of poverty and the deliberate deployment of gender disparities as a means of labor control, Harvey concludes, make the emancipation and liberation of women from their repressions a necessary condition for social change.

Analogously, the liberation of nursing—clearly a gendered profession—to disrupt the onerous male machinery of the current American health care system requires leading behaviors. The focus of my professional life swirled around primary health care as the nexus for social change, leading to equality. Over the past three decades, nurses emerged as primary care providers, trained as nurse practitioners with the toolkit to perform diagnoses and manage health problems. As nurse practitioners entered the primary care stage, they shared it with another newcomer: the physician assistant. By the beginning of the twenty-first century, four groups engaged as primary care providers (PCPs): nurse practitioners, physician assistants, allopathic physicians, and osteopathic physicians. While their education varies, their practice as PCPs is similar, focusing on integrated, accessible health care services aimed at prevention of illness as well as treatment of disease. Outcomes of all groups are available, with strong evidence that nurse practitioners provide cost-effective quality care.

Recent publications, however, address the worrisome reality of barriers erected by physicians via legislation and regulation that limit the scope of practice for nurse practitioners. As noted in the Institute of Medicine's *The Future of Nursing: Leading Change, Advancing Health*, the majority of U.S. states mandate restrictive collaborative agreements between nurse practitioners and physicians in order for nurse practitioners to practice. The collaborative agreement has become a vehicle to restrict trade, reifying physicians' power and control over reimbursement. Only seventeen states allow nurse practitioners to practice independently. Nursing leaders have historically disrupted the health delivery landscape by introducing legislation that incrementally empowered nurses with expanded scopes of practice. Even as the Institute of Medicine calls for removal of regulatory and insurance barriers to nurse practitioner practice, nursing itself must lead, disrupt, and draft amendments to nursing practice acts. Such amendments to expand the scope of practice and to remove barriers need framing in context.

Emanating from a nineteenth-century nursing model of virtue symbolized by the trope of invisibility, nursing has evolved through a tumultuous transitional period of expansion into primary care to context-based practice—an emerging heuristic. This evolving heuristic demands a new orientation to scope of practice, one deeply embedded in patient-centeredness, a perspective that broadens the definition to health to incorporate patients' priorities, be they the more traditional health issues or the less traditional ones, such as need for housing, continued education, a better job. Thus, a revisited scope of nurse practitioner PCP practice requires but a single sentence: delivery of patient-centered care is comprehensive, including the management of determinants of health within patients' living and social environments. Clearly, a disruptive definition. As broken windows are associated with urban disorder, poverty, and crime, patient-centered care is associated with an inversion of our current system: those at the bottom—patients—now calling the shots, defining what they need to consider themselves healthy. Broken windows is a powerful metaphor to describe all that rushes up behind them; so too is patient-centeredness. In 2012, the Center for Medicare and Medicaid Innovation advocated Accountable Care Organizations, groups of providers and agencies who come together to provide coordinated high-quality care to Medicare patients, receiving financial incentives for doing so. The language of patient-centeredness is entering our lexicon; the primary goal remains cost effectiveness. Beyond the recurrent themes of capitalism, however, nursing's evolving heuristic will challenge nurses and nurse practitioners alike.

What I Live For

I have lived through a time in the history of nursing in which the virtue model has receded (though not vanished), the role of nurse practitioners as primary care providers has appeared (though not with universal force), and a new heuristic model of practice based on context is just on the horizon (though not completely visible). In order for this new model to be clearer, we must follow the lead of Virginia Woolf in the last pages of *A Room of One's Own:* There is no arm to cling to, and we must go it alone. If we work for those who are to come, even though that work is deemed to be impoverished and obscure, those on whom our hopes rest will soon arrive. They will come because of our preparation.

Here is what I learned from my decisions and practice; here is how I prepared for them.

Living in borderlands is uncomfortable. A PCP, practicing under the constraints of a collaborative agreement with a physician, is neither nurse nor physician. My practice experiences vary on a continuum from a known medical model (easy and comforting) to a new heuristic nurse practitioner mode (complex and time-consuming in its socio-cognitive demands). As a nurse practitioner within the fast-track emergency service in University Hospital in Newark, I managed acute, episodic illness events, suturing and discharging with instructions for follow-up. Damn context. Whoever walked in, the patient—generally identified by his or her diagnosis—was managed on the medical model. An illness event treated. In so many ways, this practice was exciting—the rush of the emergency department—and practical, managing diagnoses rather than patients. It was also safe. If I was unsure of a diagnosis, I quickly nudged my physician colleague, defaulting to his opinion. Defaulting is easy, safe, and quick. No time spent worrying about the differential diagnoses, no need to collect more data, simply an answer delivered by the physician.

Practicing at the Mary Howard Health Center in Philadelphia was a 180-degree career switch. Here was an emerging model in which homeless patients presented with complexities in health, housing, employment, legal and welfare affairs, and family management—a population demanding more than medicine's simple lens of focusing on disease. To manage such patients while juggling realistic productivity demands against their complex holistic contexts was challenging. Thankfully, given its status as a federally qualified nurse-managed health center, Public Health Management Corporation, the owner, appreciated the value-added by the nurse practitioner approach to these complex homeless patients. While corporate management urged higher patient productivity (i.e., a daily caseload of about fifteen patients), its agents accepted lower daily figures. My patients required counseling for alternative pain management regimens, or practical how-to instructions regarding community college applications, or dietary or social work referrals: all take time, but as time increases per patient, reimbursement decreases. The focus on disease in the fast track took less time, leading to more productivity and reimbursement. The patient-centered focus took more time, leading to more referrals for lifestyle management (e.g., diet, behavioral management, social services, and health insurance). Interestingly, however, these patients return for follow-up, seeking reification for their own successful management of their lives, including their health status. Relationships with patients get established in this center, including e-mail communication with questions and concerns. In the borderland between management of illness and promotion of health, the complexities of context are enormous, requiring new webs of cognition that branch with confidence into the social and welfare systems, housing, education, and more. If accountable care organizations were to embrace context, health care by definition would move into more complex management, necessitating providers to practice at full scope, without regulatory barriers to practice.

While practice in a hospital emergency department manages illness events expediently, such practice devoid of patient context has devastating consequences, some visible and others not so. For the patient, the visit is a quick fix: the acute asthmatic bronchospasm is treated, the patient is relieved and goes home; management of his underlying respiratory hyperresponsivity is untreated, a continuing-care management plan for control of his inflammatory state unwritten. When breathless again, he will return to the hospital, the nurse practitioner treating his episodic event. Expensive illness care is again provided, without context and routine, continuing care. Shifting attention to prevention of such acute events disrupts both provider and patient. Nurse practitioner management of an asthmatic patient takes time, willingness to engage the patient and family, and attention to context (including careful identification of triggers, assessment of the home environment, and capacity to follow a daily medication regimen). Jockeying the patient to the center of the team—to lead his care management—is warranted, even if the patient is uneasy in this new role. Like nurse practitioners in transition, it is easier for patients to be told what to do rather than to control his or her own care.

Emerging to a new heuristic of context-based practice, self-efficacy is a strategic tool to bolster nurse practitioners' confidence in their domain of practice, a unique tool not borrowed from the worn leather bag of other disciplines. With patients front and center, their context visible, the primary care nurse practitioner engages in comprehensive care, keenly aware of social and environmental determinants of health.

Take Marian, a twenty-three-year-old Hispanic female, who had visited the health center initially for management of a sexually transmitted infection and acute cervicitis. With her two young children and boyfriend living with her in her elderly grandmother's apartment, Marian was quiet, extremely embarrassed by, and ashamed of, her diagnosis. When encouraged to have her boyfriend treated, she faced me squarely for the first time, stating *No!* I asked, *Are you afraid?* As she hurriedly put on her coat, I encouraged her to say no to her boyfriend, to remember Big Bird's advice: the most important person in the whole wide world is *you*! I was surprised and pleased when Marian returned two weeks later to see me, lying to the front desk that she needed a physical examination for a driver's license. Our medical assistant performed the initial steps in a physical examination—vital signs, visual acuity, height, weight, BMI—and then ushered her into an exam room. When I entered, I was thrilled to see her. *I don't need a physical exam, I already have a license,* she exclaimed. *I am scared. I am sad; my mother was bipolar and I think I am just like her!* Marian sat in the small chair adjacent to the examination table, arms folded across her chest, rocking slightly and nervously. Having been given permission to say no, Marian had two concerns: *Can I leave the father of my children? Am I crazy?* My answers surprised and relieved her. Yes to the first question, no to the second. Confident that Marian was now in charge, we designed a plan together. Marian was determined to ask her boyfriend to leave her grandmother's home, determined to obtain a restraining order to ensure her safety as well as that of her children. We went online together, Googling behavioral health services within her bus route. Finding an agency with out-patient services, Marian called and made an appointment for evaluation. While Marian's appearance was impeccable in grooming and dress, her eyes and facial expressions reflected chronic fatigue and anxiety. Uninsured but working, Marian did not have a prescription plan. I gave her a one month sample of a medication for relief of anxiety, aware that she would soon enter the behavioral health system for evaluation and management.

Facilitating Marian to meet her goals was a privilege. It took increasing confidence on my part to take the time to acknowledge context and to act on it, using context to drive interventions. At times, such interventions are quite non-traditional. The inclusion of context-based interventions is nursing's unique contribution to primary care. Acting on this contribution, however, will mandate accountability, a new self-regulation shedding codependence on the very groups that nursing historically viewed, concurrently, as both oppressors and providers—physicians and hospital administrations.

What strategies will enable the new heuristic to flourish? The scientific art of context-based practice, deeply integrating determinants of health, is an emerging body of knowledge unique to nurse practitioners; as such, nurse practitioners are not physician extenders. Self-efficacy and self-regulation will define nurse practitioners as professionals: well-educated providers with a unique conceptualization, a body of knowledge with interventions warranted in our changing health care system. Strategies surrounding self-efficacy must include firm resolve and confidence in context-based interventions. Such resolve must be balanced by evidence on the cost-effectiveness of these interventions and quality health outcomes, including patient satisfaction. Nurse practitioners themselves must provide this evidence. Increasingly, nurse practitioner education is conducted in clinical doctoral programs, with curricula immersed in research design and methodology, statistical analysis, and evidence-based practice. The faculty and students must conduct well-structured studies aimed at demonstrating efficacy of context-based, cost-effective interventions. It is not enough to teach these skills; rather, faculty must engage in them. It is no longer acceptable to simply teach evidence-based research; faculty must now practice it.

In turn, such evidence will disrupt the current coding system employed for reimbursement, the heart of the matter. Nurse practitioners must deliver evidence that context-based interventions are worthy of reimbursement by the health insurance industry. Is it, in fact, less expensive to manage health than to manage illness? Shifting this giant from an illness model (medicine's orientation) to a health model (nurse practitioner's orientation) is a herculean task whose onus has been felt by both the Clinton and Obama administrations. Nurse practitioners cannot abrogate this responsibility to others when it comes to demonstrating the efficacy of their care model. We must emerge from the fog of hybridity as leaders.

Tactically, nurse practitioners must pursue collaborators and align to become a more powerful force for negotiating health insurance contracts, reimbursement rates, and privileging. State nurse practitioner organizations, nurse practitioner coalitions, the National Nursing Centers Consortium, and other similar groups provide validation, structure, and potential for replication of models through efficiency in cluster demonstration grants. In absence of leadership among nurse practitioners, other disciplines may determine the fate of context-based interventions. Emerging from invisible practice in middle earth, nurse practitioners must align as the lead agents in efforts financially sponsored by large foundations (such as the Robert Wood Johnson Foundation) and validated by institutions (such as the Institute of Medicine).

Self-regulation strategies require dismissal of value dualisms and acts of defiance. In that nursing grew as a profession by the route of legislation rather than through the more standard avenue of higher education, the embrace of amendments to nursing practice acts is now needed. Crafting amendments to nursing legislation that remove barriers imposed by medicine on nurse practitioner practice is the responsibility of nurse practitioners. Rather than living in the secure but unpleasant borderlands between medicine and nursing, nurse practitioners must resolve to work with legislators to introduce liberating language in nursing legislation. Such disruption will require courage based on confidence in our educational programs and evidence-based practice. For tactics, nurse practitioners must learn effective political activism, including lobbying techniques, negotiation and compromise, and regulatory reform. These processes take time, requiring a long view of success. Nurse practitioners must initiate, sustain, and promote these tactics. In this period during which a new heuristic is being framed, daily practice and legislative action must be interrelated. The nurse practitioner student must be expected to pursue knowledge of therapeutic lifestyle management. The allure of cure, the drama of acute illness management—helicopters hovering above a hospital heliport—must be exchanged for the context-based interventions taking time, patient (and provider) self-discipline, and more socially just models of reimbursement. Both student and seasoned nurse practitioner must appreciate that legislative change takes time, is incremental, and depends on strongly validated practices. Nurse practitioners must be bricoleurs—tenacious and resilient—to evolve as functional members of the new heuristic of context-based primary care.

I began this book with allusion to Robert Frost's "The Road Not Taken" and end it with reference to Henry David Thoreau's *Walden*. The moral conscience of our nation, Thoreau wrote about looking down to look up. My left side became unsteady after my stroke, and I follow my feet. I see puddles in the city. I see tide pools at the ocean. I see the sandy bottom and know the shallowness of it all. I know all about how the thin current slides away, and I know how eternity remains.

Spring

To document my life, I have written this book as a woman and a nurse.

From a traditional virtue script for nursing to a context-driven nurse practitioner model, my career has been accompanied by change. Some of it I witnessed, and some of it I caused. I have emerged from the fog of hybridity. The risks I have experienced shake me to my core. The gains are breathtaking. For whom have the chances been taken?

Think of Cynthia, my tall, thin, 160-pound, sixty-year-old African American female patient. You will remember her flat and expressionless affect. You will recall her hypertension and anemia.

Do you hear voices? she asked.

Yes, I did.

How different are blacks and whites? she asked. *We are alike, right?*

Yes, we are alike. All of us are alike.

Index

About the Author

Frances Ward, former David R. Devereaux chair of nursing and professor emerita at Temple University College of Health Professions and Social Work, has extensive experience in higher education, academic administration, and clinical practice. As founding dean of the school of nursing at the University of Medicine and Dentistry of New Jersey, she established articulated undergraduate and graduate programs, launching an interdisciplinary doctoral program in urban systems. Deeply committed to quality health care delivery for urban residents, she currently serves as a part-time adult nurse practitioner at a nurse-managed health center. Her research, focusing on issues integral to care delivery among uninsured and underinsured populations, evolves from her practice. She has received grants from the Hearst Foundation and the Robert Wood Johnson Foundation to support her urban health efforts. Emphasizing the value of advanced practice nurses in primary care, she has been integral in legislative efforts solidifying scope of practice gains for nurse practitioners. Her book *On Duty: Power, Politics, and the History of Nursing in New Jersey* was published by Rutgers University Press in 2009.